Keyla Jiménez
Henry Suárez
Iskra Suárez

Prevalence of the degree of hyponatremia in patients with liver cirrhosis.

Keyla Jiménez
Henry Suárez
Iskra Suárez

Prevalence of the degree of hyponatremia in patients with liver cirrhosis.

Degree of hyponatremia in patients with liver cirrhosis admitted to the gastroenterology department of a public hospital.

ScienciaScripts

Imprint

Any brand names and product names mentioned in this book are subject to trademark, brand or patent protection and are trademarks or registered trademarks of their respective holders. The use of brand names, product names, common names, trade names, product descriptions etc. even without a particular marking in this work is in no way to be construed to mean that such names may be regarded as unrestricted in respect of trademark and brand protection legislation and could thus be used by anyone.

Cover image: www.ingimage.com

This book is a translation from the original published under ISBN 978-613-9-46666-5.

Publisher:
Sciencia Scripts
is a trademark of
Dodo Books Indian Ocean Ltd. and OmniScriptum S.R.L publishing group

120 High Road, East Finchley, London, N2 9ED, United Kingdom
Str. Armeneasca 28/1, office 1, Chisinau MD-2012, Republic of Moldova, Europe
Printed at: see last page
ISBN: 978-620-8-32882-5

Copyright © Keyla Jiménez, Henry Suárez, Iskra Suárez
Copyright © 2024 Dodo Books Indian Ocean Ltd. and OmniScriptum S.R.L publishing group

GENERAL INDEX

SUMMARY

Introduction: *Hyponatremia is a hydroelectrolyte disturbance defined as a serum sodium concentration of less than 135 mEq/L or 135 mmol/L, being the most frequent electrolyte imbalance in clinical practice; in patients with cirrhosis, hyponatremia is considered when serum sodium is less than 130 mEq/L.* ***Objective: To*** *estimate the prevalence of degrees of hyponatremia in patients with liver cirrhosis admitted to the gastroenterology department of the Hospital General del Norte de Guayaquil IESS Los Ceibos between January 2021 and June 2022.* ***Methodology:*** *The study was observational, retrospective, cross-sectional, descriptive; a sample of 111 patients whose information was obtained from medical records was analysed.* ***Results:*** *The predominance of female sex (50.5%) was identified, as well as age between 51 and 70 years (64.9%); 63.1% used diuretics and 72.1% had a hospital stay of 1 to 15 days. It was also identified that mild hyponatraemia had a prevalence of 23.7%, moderate hyponatraemia a rate of 10.1% and severe hyponatraemia a rate of 1.3%. Regarding comorbidities, cancer was the only comorbidity related to hyponatraemia levels (sig. 0.049 < 0.05), being mostly at the moderate level. Most patients had decompensated cirrhosis (80.2%), where 51.4% were in the mild hyponatraemia grade. On the other hand, ADH was the only complication related to the degree of hyponatraemia (sig. 0.032 < 0.05), with 23.4% with mild hyponatraemia.* ***Conclusion:*** *We conclude that the prevalence of hyponatraemia in patients with cirrhosis overall was 35.1%.*

Keywords: *Prevalence, hyponatraemia, degree of hyponatraemia, liver cirrhosis, clinical stage of cirrhosis.*

INTRODUCTION

Cirrhosis is a disease with a major public health impact that should be considered of great concern. In recent years the trend has shown a slight increase worldwide (1).According to the exploration of the results of the Global Burden of Disease 2019 study, it is estimated that this pathology caused 1,472,011.82 deaths worldwide, which represents 2.60% of deaths during that year (2).In the USA, 5.5 million people (representing 2% of the US population) have been diagnosed with cirrhosis, the seventh leading cause of death in the country (3).In Ecuador, according to data from the National Institute of Statistics and Census 2021, cirrhosis of the liver ranks 85th on the list of morbidities. With respect to mortality, this pathology has decreased compared to other years. It ranks 10th among the 10 leading causes of death with 2,481 people, representing 2.4%. Cirrhosis in men and women is ranked 9th, with 2.4% and 1.9%, respectively (4).Liver cirrhosis is the final stage of chronic liver damage, and is characterised by fibrosis leading to distortion of the normal liver architecture with destruction of functional tissue, being replaced by nodular tissue without complete recovery of liver function, which can lead to various complications such as portal hypertension (oesophageal varices, ascites), with the possibility of progression to hepatocarcinoma, liver failure or death (5).The pathophysiology of liver cirrhosis, regardless of the aetiology, is produced by a repair reaction in response to damage and inflammation mediated by inflammatory agents (interleukins, cytokines, etc.) producing anatomopathological changes in the hepatocyte, as well as altering the hepatic microvasculature. (angiogenesis, endothelial dysfunction, sinusoidal remodelling and intrahepatic shunt formation) (5).These changes in liver structure lead to disturbances of normal liver function such as portal hypertension, alterations of the liver profile (hyperbilirubinaemia, thrombocytopenia and reduced production of coagulation factors), hypoalbuminaemia and electrolyte disturbances such as hyponatraemia (6). Hyponatraemia is a water-electrolyte disturbance defined as a serum sodium concentration of less than 135 mEq/L or 135 mmol/L, and is the most common electrolyte imbalance in clinical practice, occurring in 15% to 30% of hospitalised patients (7).In patients with cirrhosis, hyponatraemia is considered hyponatraemia when serum sodium is less than 130 mEq/L. Hyponatraemia in cirrhotic patients can be hypervolaemic or dilutional, hypovolaemic or normovolaemic (hypervolaemic is the most common), and its pathophysiology is complex because it involves splanchnic vasodilation, resulting in activation of ADH (antidiuretic hormone) by the renin-angiotensin-aldosterone system

(RAAS), which allows exaggerated reabsorption of water volumes, with a subsequent relative excess of total body water and the development of dilutional hyponatraemia (8).The clinical picture of hyponatraemia is often non-specific and may include nausea and/or vomiting, anorexia, sensory disturbances (confusion to coma), gait disturbances, severe headaches, and even death. Several studies have shown that cirrhotic patients with hyponatraemia have an impact on quality of life, frequent hospitalisations, increased morbidity and mortality and incidence of cirrhosis-related complications such as refractory ascites, upper gastrointestinal bleeding, spontaneous bacterial peritonitis and hepatic encephalopathy, especially considering the relationship of the degree of hyponatraemia (8) (9).

CHAPTER I
PROBLEM STATEMENT

1.1. PROBLEM STATEMENT

This study consists of estimating the prevalence of the degree of hyponatremia in patients with liver cirrhosis in the Gastroenterology service of the Hospital General del Norte de Guayaquil IESS Los Ceibos in the period from January 2021 to June 2022.

In our setting, there is no record of up-to-date research on the prevalence of the degree of hyponatraemia in patients with liver cirrhosis. It is essential to take into account the degree of hyponatraemia in order to define the severity and possible complications that may occur in patients with liver cirrhosis. Our study would provide health personnel with knowledge on various aspects of hyponatraemia in liver cirrhosis: clinical and complementary examinations, pathophysiology and associated complications in our environment (e.g. ascites, hepatic encephalopathy, among others), avoiding an increase in morbidity and mortality in this population and reducing public health spending.

1.2. GENERAL OBJECTIVE

To estimate the prevalence of hyponatremia in patients with liver cirrhosis admitted to the Gastroenterology Department of the Hospital General del Norte de Guayaquil IESS Los Ceibos between January 2021 and June 2022.

1.3. SPECIFIC OBJECTIVES

1. Relate the degree of hyponatraemia to comorbidities associated with liver cirrhosis.

2. To correlate the severity of cirrhosis according to the Child-Pugh scale and the degree of hyponatraemia in the patients to be studied.

3. To identify the clinical stage of cirrhosis (compensated or uncompensated) in which the different degrees of hyponatraemia occur most frequently in the population studied.

4. To determine the relationship between the degree of hyponatraemia and the most frequent complications in patients with liver cirrhosis (ascites, hepatic encephalopathy, upper gastrointestinal haemorrhage).

1.4. RESEARCH VARIABLES

Table 1. Operationalisation of variables

Name Variables	Definition of the variable	Type	Value final
Hyponatraemia	Serum sodium level < 135 mEq/L	Nominal categorical dichotomous	Yes/No
Degree of hyponatremia	Mild: <130 - 135 mEq/L. Moderate: 125 - 129 mEq/L. Severe: <125 mEq/L	Categorical ordinal polytomous	Mild, Moderate, Severe
Age	Number of years	Numeric discreet	Number of years
Sex	Patient phenotype	Nominal categorical dichotomous	Female / Male
Drugs	Use of diuretics	Nominal categorical dichotomous	Yes/No
Associated comorbidity	Concomitant diseases disorder to be studied	Nominal categorical polytomics	Hypertension Arterial hypertension; Diabetes Mellitus; Kidney disease chronicle; Cancer; Infectious (Tubercle sis)
Ascites	Presence of fluid in peritoneal cavity	Nominal categorical dichotomous	Yes/No
Clinical stage of cirrhosis	Stage of the disease	Categorical nominal dichotomous	Compensates da / Decompensada

Duration of the hospital stay	Number of days hospitalised	Numeric discreet	Number of days
Child-Pugh Scale	Severity classification of the liver cirrhosis	Categorical ordinal polytomics	A, B or C
Hepatic encephalopathy	Presence of hepatic encephalopathy	Nominal categorical dichotomous	Yes/No
Oesophageal varices	Presence of oesophageal varices without bleeding	Categorical dichotomous	Yes/No
Upper gastrointestinal bleeding of variceal origin	Active bleeding from oesophageal varices	Categorical dichotomous	Yes/No
Jaundice	Presence of yellowish discolouration of the skin and of mucous membranes	Categorical dichotomous	Yes/No

1.5.JUSTIFICATION OF THE PROBLEM

Liver cirrhosis is considered a public health problem affecting the general population due to increased morbidity and mortality, as well as higher economic costs and an impact on the patient's quality of life, together with deficiencies in research and statistical data collection for the development of prevention and treatment measures for this pathology.

On the other hand, water and electrolyte disturbances, such as hyponatraemia, have been shown to be a predictor of morbidity and mortality in cirrhotic patients, and it has been observed that this disturbance occurs more frequently in patients with decompensated liver cirrhosis, but in other cases it can occur asymptomatically in stable cirrhotic patients, so early detection would imply adequate therapy for the prevention of long-term complications.

In the Hospital General Norte de Guayaquil IESS Los Ceibos there have been no studies on the degree of hyponatremia in patients with liver cirrhosis, so it is considered necessary to develop one to know the epidemiological picture of this water and electrolyte disorder.

In order to carry out this study, we have the availability of time, financial, material and patient resources. Secondary data will be used by means of the documentation technique, in which a review of clinical histories in the hospitalisation area of Gastroenterology at the Hospital General Norte de Guayaquil IESS Los Ceibos will be carried out with the appropriate authorisation and which meet the required inclusion criteria, together with the collection and analysis of the variables to be studied to estimate the prevalence of the degree of hyponatremia in patients with liver cirrhosis admitted to the Gastroenterology area of the Hospital General del Norte de Guayaquil IESS Los Ceibos in the period from January 2021 to June 2022.

CHAPTER II
THEORETICAL FRAMEWORK

2.1. LIVER CIRRHOSIS

2.1.1. DEFINITION

Liver cirrhosis, with its variety and regardless of its aetiology, is established as a chronic, progressive and irreversible pathological condition present in the final stage of liver fibrosis, with the particularity of forming regeneration nodules, destroying the normal hepatic anatomy and damaging its physiology, leading to serious complications that affect the quality of life of the cirrhotic patient (5).

2.1.2. AETIOLOGY AND RISK FACTORS FOR LIVER CIRRHOSIS

Liver cirrhosis has a wide variety of aetiologies, which in turn can be considered as implicit risk factors. Among the main and most frequent are cirrhosis of alcoholic origin, cirrhosis of viral origin (Hepatitis B and Hepatitis C), and non-alcoholic fatty liver disease. In addition, less frequent causes include cirrhosis due to autoimmune hepatitis, drug-induced cirrhosis, vascular disorders, storage diseases such as haemochromatosis, Wilson's disease and alpha-1 antitrypsin deficiency. Each aetiology will be briefly described below (6):

a. Alcoholic cirrhosis: Excessive ethanol consumption promotes the production of free radicals that contribute to the functional failure of liver cells and the release of cytokines, leading to the destruction of hepatocytes (10).

b. Cirrhosis of viral aetiology: This is caused by infection with hepatitis B and C viruses. According to PAHO, 57% of patients diagnosed with liver cirrhosis are of viral origin, specifically HBV and HCV (11). A descriptive study conducted in Cuba by Corrales et al. in 2021 mentions that more than 350 million people around the world are considered chronic carriers of the B virus surface antigen, DNA virus, and of this group, more than half are considered chronic carriers of hepatitis B virus surface antigen, DNA virus, and of this group, more than half are considered chronic carriers of hepatitis B virus surface antigen, DNA virus.only 15-30% may develop liver failure, cirrhosis and even hepatocellular carcinoma. With regard to patients infected with HCV, an RNA virus, this represents very alarming numbers of cases diagnosed with cirrhosis due to this virus (12).

c. Cirrhosis due to NASH (non-alcoholic steatohepatitis): Non-alcoholic steatohepatitis is the presence of injury at the hepatocellular level, not preceded by excessive alcohol consumption, but as a multifactorial process involving hygienic-dietary factors. Although the exact pathophysiology is not known, the current prevailing theory is the phenomenon of "lipotoxicity" leading to an accelerated scarring process, the development of a degree of fibrosis and progression to cirrhosis (13).

d. Cirrhosis due to autoimmune hepatitis: This is the hepatitis that occurs in patients with a greater genetic predisposition, in which the immune system is responsible for destroying the hepatocytes, causing chronic, definitive and severe damage. The female population has a greater tendency to suffer from it, considering the existence of an immunomodulator gene on the X chromosome or the possibility of the effect of oestrogens and some sex hormones that may influence antigen recognition (14).

e. Drug-induced cirrhosis: Drug-induced liver toxicity may be asymptomatic and may be an incidental finding in laboratory tests, while symptomatic liver toxicity may show evidence of liver failure. The drugs that can cause liver cirrhosis are very varied, but the following are recognised: analgesics (NSAIDs), certain antibiotics (fluoroquinolones, macrolides, etc.), antituberculosis drugs such as isoniazid, antiarrhythmics such as amiodarone, immunomodulators (azathioprine), among others (15). It should be remembered that drug-induced liver cirrhosis is based on four important concepts: chronic use or abuse of the drug, the pattern of hepatic injury (hepatocellular injury, cholestatic or mixed), risk factors (age, race, gender, pregnancy, alcohol consumption, comorbidities and genetics) and drug-associated factors (metabolism and lipophilicity) (16).

2.1.3. PATHOPHYSIOLOGY OF LIVER CIRRHOSIS

Liver cirrhosis is characterised by a history of chronic parenchymal injury, persistent activation of various inflammatory mediators and an uncontrolled scarring process. Liver fibrogenesis is a distinctly dynamic process, involving biomolecular processes that result in an exaggerated accumulation of extracellular matrix components (collagen type I, II and IV, fibronectin and laminin proteoglycans) in the liver parenchyma produced by activated myofibroblasts, cells differentiated from "hepatic stellate cells" (perisinusoidal quiescent cells), responsible for modulating the immunomodulatory response and angiogenesis (17).

The importance of stellate cells in the pathophysiology of liver cirrhosis, which originate from the transdifferentiation of these stellate cells into activated ECM-producing myofibroblasts, should be detailed, and which are activated by hepatocyte apoptosis from a biochemical signal (DAMPs or Damage-associated patterns), the most studied for its role in the pathogenesis of liver cirrhosis being HMGB1, together with the recruitment of immune cells such as Kupffer cells, T-lymphocytes, and monocytes, which secrete immune cells such as Kupffer cells, T-lymphocytes, and monocytes. and monocytes, which secrete proinflammatory cytokines (18).

Physiologically, this fibrogenesis process is controlled by anti-fibrotic mechanisms that prevent the formation of regenerative nodules; but in the development of cirrhosis, the activation and ECM production of stellate cells persists, together with the appearance of free radicals, cytokines and chemokines, favouring a pro-fibrogenic and pro-angiogenic microenvironment (17) (18).The term cirrhosis is associated with a change in liver microanatomy, in which regenerative parenchymal nodules surrounded by fibrous septa and changes in vascular architecture occur, resulting in altered pressure gradients of the splanchnic portal vascular system, with the development of portal hypertension and its consequences (variceal gastrointestinal bleeding, hepatic encephalopathy, ascites, hepatorenal syndrome, etc.) and an increased risk of hepatocellular carcinoma (17).

Portal hypertension in liver cirrhosis arises from hepatic vessel obstruction due to hepatic structural changes and altered portal vascular tone, vascular obliteration and increased intrahepatic vascular resistance due to fibrogenesis. In addition to the following pathophysiological mechanisms (19):

• A reduction in the bioavailability of nitric oxide.

• Potent vasoconstrictors (ET-1, prostaglandin H2, thromboxane A2, and leukotrienes).
• Splanchnic hyperflow due to vasodilators (Angiotensin 1-7, endogenous cannabinoids and carbon monoxide).
• Hypocontractility vascular intrinsic y formation of portosystemic collaterals by pro-angiogenic factors (VEGF and PDGF).

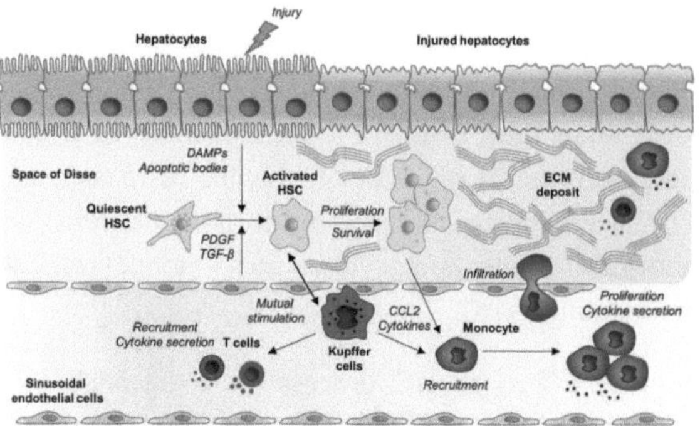

Note: Chronic hepatocyte injury results in the release of Damage-associated patterns (DAMPs) and apoptotic cells that activate hepatic stellate cells (HSCs) and the recruitment of immune cells. Complex multidirectional interactions between HSCs and immune cells promote transdifferentiation of extracellular matrix (ECM)-producing fibroblasts. PDGF: platelet growth-activating factor; TGF-B: growth factor beta; CCL2: chemokine chemokine ligand 2: Roehlen N, Crouchet E, Baumert TF. Liver Fibrosis: Mechanistic Concepts and Therapeutic Perspectives. Cells [Internet]. April 2020 [cited 2022 Oct 26];9(4):875. Available from: https://www.mdpi.com/2073-4409/9/4/875

2.1.4. MANIFESTATIONS CLINICS Y STAGES CLINICAL OF LIVER CIRRHOSIS

Liver cirrhosis can present asymptomatically or symptomatically, depending on whether compensated or decompensated cirrhosis is present. Compensated cirrhosis usually presents asymptomatically, and is an incidental finding in laboratory tests (elevated aminotransferases or GGT), physical examination (hepatomegaly or splenomegaly) or imaging (ultrasound with signs of liver cirrhosis); whereas in decompensated cirrhosis the patient presents with a plethora of signs and symptoms (20).The clinical manifestations of liver cirrhosis can be divided according to the system affected, which are presented below (21):

1) **Gastrointestinal system:** Portal hypertension via portosystemic collaterals leads to ascites, hepatosplenomegaly, prominent abdominal umbilical veins (caput medusae or medusa head) and upper gastrointestinal bleeding from oesophageal varices. In cirrhosis of alcoholic origin, there is an increased risk of

acute pancreatitis, bacterial overgrowth and cholelithiasis/cholecystitis.

2) Lymphohaematopoietic system: Anaemia may occur in cirrhotic patients due to folate depletion, haemolysis (in alcoholic cirrhosis), pancytopenia due to hypersplenism and alteration of coagulation factors (PT and TTP), with possible complications such as PTE, DVT, AMI, stroke and disseminated intravascular coagulation (DIC).

3) Renal system: Portal hypertension produces a state of renal hypoperfusion, resulting in a hepatorenal syndrome induced by persistent activation of the renin-angiotensin-aldosterone system (RAAS) for sodium and water retention, and renal vasoconstriction in an attempt to overcome systemic vasodilatation.

4) Pulmonary system: Pulmonary manifestations of cirrhosis are oxygen desaturation, ventilation/perfusion mismatch (V/Q mismatch), reduced pulmonary diffusing capacity and hyperventilation. Less common: hepatopulmonary syndrome, portopulmonary hypertension, hepatic hydrothorax,

5) Integumentary system: Cutaneous manifestations such as jaundice, pruritus, lichen simplex chronicus, spider angiomas, telangiectasias and palmar erythema. In addition, finger changes such as hypocratism, osteoarthropathy, Dupuytren's contracture, Terry's nails and Muehrcke's lines have been documented.

6) Endocrine system: Cirrhotic patients often develop gynaecomastia, hypogonadism, and in women amenorrhoea, infertility and irregular menstrual bleeding may occur.Other clinical manifestations that have been identified on physical examination are hepatic stench (mouldy, faecal breath produced by accumulation of ketones and mercaptans) and asterixis (fluttering tremor on extension and dorsiflexion) (21).

2.1.4.1. UPPER GASTROINTESTINAL BLEEDING OF VARICEAL ORIGIN

Gastrointestinal bleeding is defined as bleeding above the ligament of Treitz. Portal hypertension stands out as the main cause for the development of future complications of liver cirrhosis such as: oesophageal varices formation, ascites, alteration of coagulation factors, hepatorenal syndrome, heart disease and some pulmonary complications.In a compensated clinical stage, oesophageal varices will not show symptoms and tend to be benign, but depending on the changes in venous portal pressure, variceal bleeding or rebleeding may occur. In decompensated cirrhosis, they are characterised by haemorrhagic oesophageal varices that complicate the picture, and upper endoscopic video endoscopy (VEDA) is of great diagnostic and therapeutic use.Endoscopic intervention is recommended within 24 hours of hospital admission, and classification into low-risk and high-risk oesophageal varices; but other non-invasive diagnostic means such as echoendoscopy, elastography, capsule endoscopy and other imaging studies (tomography and magnetic resonance imaging) are recommended (22) (23).

Graph 2. Relationship between portal venous pressure and the risk of developing oesophageal varices and upper gastrointestinal bleeding.

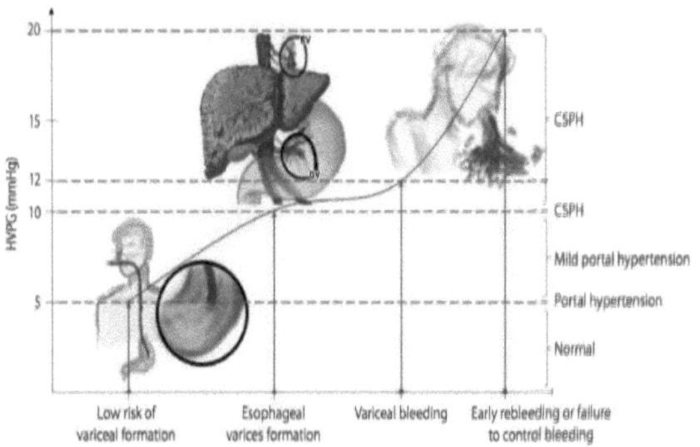

There are two important scales to assess upper gastrointestinal bleeding in cirrhotics: the Glasgow-Blatchford Score (GBS) and the Rockall Score (RS), which help us to predict adverse outcomes in a specific period and the ideal time for intervention (24).Both scales can be used as they have an equivalent positive predictive value, but they are not in everyday use due to their limitations and complexity factors: the GBS requires the reporting of data on chronic diseases and comorbidities of the patient while the RS requires a mandatory endoscopic diagnosis to perform the calculation (25).

2.1.4.2. DECOMPENSATED LIVER CIRRHOSIS

Decompensation of liver cirrhosis develops from several pathophysiological scenarios that occur together for the development of liver cirrhosis, such as (26):

1. Portal hypertension (hepatic venous pressure gradient >10 mmhg) and formation of portosystemic collaterals by activation of VEGF (vascular endothelial growth factor).
2. hyperdynamic circulation (ascites, hyponatraemia, HD and other complications of liver cirrhosis)

3. Translocation of bacterial endotoxins and elevated levels of pro-inflammatory mediators (angiotensin II, noradrenaline, TNF-alpha, IL-3, IL-6 and IL-33 receptor).

4. Mitochondrial collapse and oxidative damage, apoptosis and local tissue dysfunction, inflammasome-mediated cytokine storm (e.g. NLRP3) and histone-free mitochondrial DNA (mtDNA) for propagation of cell damage to distant organs.

ASCITES IN LIVER CIRRHOSIS

Ascites in liver cirrhosis is defined as the accumulation of fluid in the peritoneal cavity, assessable on physical examination as significant abdominal distension or by ultrasound, which can be classified according to its severity: grade 1, grade 2 and grade 3 (tension ascites). The occurrence of ascites has been shown to be a poor prognostic factor in patients with liver cirrhosis, and usually follows upper gastrointestinal bleeding of variceal origin.Ascites is multifactorial in origin and several hypotheses have been proposed for its development, one of which mentions peripheral and splanchnic arterial vasodilatation together with activation of several neurohormonal pathways leading to renal dysfunction with water and sodium retention and decreased glomerular filtration rate (27). Classically, the process of ascites is divided into 5 phases occurring at different time intervals: a **pre-ascitic phase** (hyperdynamic circulation and increased cardiac output), a **second phase** (reduced natriuresis even with ADH action), a **third phase** (sodium retention by RAAS and SNS due to progressive splanchnic arterial vasodilatation), a **fourth phase** (reduced GFR and renal perfusion) and a **fifth** phase (onset of type 1 or type 2 Hepatorenal Syndrome) (27) (28) .

2.1.4.3.   ICTERICIA

Jaundice is the clinical manifestation of hyperbilirubinaemia, and is defined as yellowing of the skin, mucous membranes and conjunctivae, with the threshold serum value being greater than 3 g/dl of serum bilirubin. Jaundice usually occurs in the later stages of liver cirrhosis, accompanied by other stigmata of chronic liver disease or in an underlying malignant cause associated with liver cirrhosis such as pancreatic head cancer (29).Diagnosis is clinical and based on laboratory tests such as liver function tests, serum bilirubin, hepatocellular profile (viral serology, antibodies, etc.).autoimmune) and cholestatic studies such as abdominal ultrasound, computed tomography, magnetic resonance imaging, retrograde cholangiopancreatography (ERCP), percutaneous transhepatic cholangiography (PTTC) and endoscopic ultrasound (29).There are several aetiologies that can cause jaundice, classified as **conjugated hyperbilirubinaemia** (genetic syndromes such as: hepatocellular disease such as hepatitis A-B-C, extrahepatic biliary obstruction such as choledocholithiasis, Dubin-Jhonson Syndrome and Rotor Syndrome, and neoplasms), **unconjugated hyperbilirubinaemia** (haemolytic anaemias, Gilbert's Syndrome, Crigler-Najjar syndrome type 1 and 2, hyperthyroidism and hyperestrogenism), **mixed hyperbilirubinaemia** and **pseudoictericia** (Addison's disease, use of suntan lotions, hypercarotinaemia and certain drugs such as rifabutin) (30).

2.1.4.4. HEPATIC ENCEPHALOPATHY

Hepatic encephalopathy (HE) is a complex neurological syndrome caused by hepatic failure and/or portosystemic short circuits, manifesting as a broad spectrum of neurological, musculoskeletal and psychiatric abnormalities, ranging from subclinical alterations to coma. HD causes significant morbidity and mortality.In asymptomatic patients, HD can be detected by means of specialised tests designed to uncover subtle changes in the patient's mental state; these include psychometric tests of attention, working memory and learning, psychomotor speed and visuospatial ability (Psychometric Hepatic Encephalopathy Score (PHES), Portosystemic Encephalopathy Syndrome (PES) test in minimal or subclinical HD, The Block Design Test, SCAN Test and the Stroop App Test) (31).These tests have been shown to have high sensitivity and low cost. It presents certain limitations such as time, the need for trained staff and variability of results according to patient age and education (32).

2.1.4.4.1. PATHOPHYSIOLOGY

At present, the pathophysiology of HD has not yet been established. Neurotoxic levels of ammonium are thought to be developmentally involved, exerting their neurotoxic action through cellular oedema, inflammation, oxidative stress, mitochondrial dysfunction, disruption of cellular bioenergetics, changes in pH and altered membrane potential. No direct correlation has been demonstrated between the severity of HD and the degree of hyperammonaemia but it has been clarified that a diagnosis of HD is incompatible with normal ammonaemia levels (33).Other pathophysiological alterations that have been studied in the development of HD include(33) (34) (35) (36) (37):

- Oxidative stress (neuroinflammation and blood-brain barrier dysfunction).
- Bile acids (proliferation of urease-producing bacteria).

● Alteration of minerals such as manganese and zinc, dilutional hyponatraemia).

● Neuropathological changes (astrocyte oedema and neuronal death due to senescence).

● Disruption of the microbiota-liver-brain axis (bacterial translocation and neuroinflammation by endotoxins) and malnutrition (muscle hypercatabolism, thiamine and B12 deficiency and sarcopenia).

● Inhibitory neurotransmitters (gamma-aminobutyric acid or GABA) and transjugular intrahepatic portosystemic shunt (TIPS) in the treatment of liver cirrhosis.

Figure 3. Role of the gut-brain axis in hepatic encephalopathy.

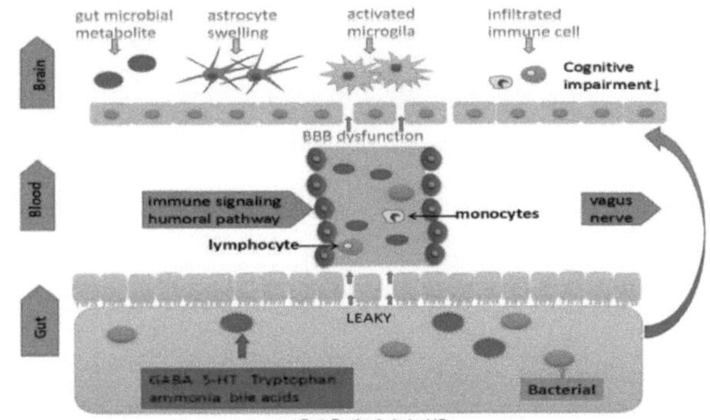

2.1.4.4.2. CLINICAL MANIFESTATIONS

In the earliest stages, patients usually report mild symptoms, such as sleep-wake cycle disturbance (sleepwalking, drowsiness); with progression to abrupt personality changes such as apathy, irritability, disinhibition, and finally neurocognitive disturbances such as disorientation, dysarthria, confusion and eventually coma (32) (34) .

Hepatic encephalopathy also affects the musculoskeletal system, with asterixis being the most characteristic but not pathognomonic sign, produced by hyperextension of the wrists on extension of the arms, resulting in a sudden and repetitive drooping (like the wings of a bird); it can also be seen in the lower limbs, arms, tongue and eyelids (34).Other musculoskeletal manifestations are hyperreflexia, clonus, muscle rigidity, and specifically in cirrhotic patients an irreversible pseudoparkinsonian syndrome may occur, resulting in extrapyramidal symptoms such as hypomimia (reduced facial expressivity), rigidity, bradykinesia, bradykinesia, bradypsychia and parkinsonian tremors (32).

2.1.4.4.3. CLASSIFICATION

HD is categorised based on 4 characteristics: the underlying disease, the severity of manifestations, the time course of symptomatology (episodic, recurrent if occurring at intervals of 6 months or less or persistent), and whether there are precipitating factors (infections, gastrointestinal bleeding, diuretic use, water-electrolyte abnormalities and constipation) (32).

The first categorisation criterion is the underlying disease, which allows HD to be subdivided into 3 types: type A hepatic encephalopathy (in acute liver failure), type B (present in portosystemic shunts) and type C (the most frequent and most common type of hepatic encephalopathy).present in liver cirrhosis or a portosystemic shunt with liver dysfunction. and is associated with other signs of chronic liver disease (38).

To classify severity, patients are graded using the West Haven Criteria, which starts from minimal HD (Grade 0) to Grade IV, taking into consideration the clinical manifestations of HD and the patient's mental status according to the Glasgow Coma Scale (32).The degrees of Hepatic Encephalopathy according to the West Haven Scale are plotted in the following chart:

Table 2. Grades of Hepatic Encephalopathy

Degree of hepatic encephalopathy	Clinical manifestations
Grade 0 (minimal or subclinical)	Abnormal results in psychometric or neurophysiological tests, but without symptomatology.
Grade I	Personality changes, with mild confusion, dysarthria and alterations in sleep patterns (insomnia, sleepwalking, etc.).
Grade II	Lethargy and/or apathy, dysarthria, disinhibition, disorientation, dyspraxia and asterixis.
Grade III	Drowsiness to stupor, confusion, bizarre behaviour and temporo-spatial disorientation. Possible decortication or decerebration.
Grade IV	Coma and opisthotonos.

A major limitation of the West Haven classification is the inter-observer and intra-observer variability in its use, which is explained by the interpretation of symptomatology and the ability to detect subtle changes in patient behaviour, resulting in subjectivity and imprecision in differentiating between early and late HD (31).

2.1.4.4.4. DIAGNOSIS

Diagnosis is based on clinical judgement and the severity of the disease by means of the Child-Pugh or MELD scale, in order to rule out other causes of neuropsychiatric disease and to initiate early treatment according to the following points (33) (38) (39):

• Neuropsychiatric profiling using standardised and specialised tests. Use Glasgow Coma Scale in uncooperative patients.

• Nutritional history and assessment of nutritional status.
• Identification of HD episodes, precipitants and whether they required hospitalisation.
• Laboratory tests such as blood biometry, liver and kidney function, electrolytes, TSH, CRP, glycaemia, vitamin B12 and urinalysis to rule out other aetiologies of encephalopathy.

• Imaging tests, indicated if the patient's symptoms are unusual, the onset of symptoms is abrupt or severe, manifestation of focal neurological signs or limited or no response to treatment. Imaging may include: computed tomography, positron emission computed tomography, magnetic resonance imaging (T1, T2-FLAIR, DWI, ADC, etc.), electroencephalogram (EEG) and ultimately anatomopathological study of the brain biopsy.

• Assessment of response to treatment of precipitating factors or hypoammonemic strategies.

Ammonium levels are currently not considered as a screening test for HD diagnosis as they are unreliable due to certain limitations, such as: hyperammonaemia in other clinical situations (urease-producing bacterial UTI, gastrointestinal bleeding, renal disease, portosystemic shunt, nutrition, etc.). parenteral, salicylate, drug and alcohol intoxication) or poor blood sample collection and storage (39).

2.1.5.COMPLEMENTARY STUDIES FOR THE DIAGNOSIS OF LIVER CIRRHOSIS

The diagnosis of liver cirrhosis is clinical, but it is still necessary to resort to validated complementary studies that have demonstrated validity for the definitive diagnosis of liver cirrhosis, with liver biopsy currently considered the gold standard, but with certain disadvantages: cost, invasive technique and poor biopsy technique.

Before resorting to liver biopsy, use should be made of scales, formulas and imaging tests that have been shown to be diagnostically useful, cost-effective, non-invasive and can be applied repeatedly. The imaging studies used to assess the degree of fibrosis and cirrhosis are ultrasound, computed tomography and magnetic resonance imaging, but they have a low to moderate diagnostic accuracy for identifying cirrhosis, and currently liver elastography (FibroScan) has become the non-invasive method of choice for quantifying liver stiffness (elasticity) (40) (41).

- **Ultrasound:** Detects the development of portal hypertension, splenomegaly and ascites by colour Doppler. FibroScan currently allows assessment of reduced hepatic elasticity or increased stiffness in kilopascals or metres per second, and other modalities such as ARFI and 2D-SWE are available for more accurate measurement.
- **Computed tomography: This** allows us to visualise morphological liver changes, signs of cirrhosis and portal hypertension such as splenomegaly, collateral venous circulation and portal vein thickening; and other techniques such as perfusion CT and Fibro-CT (chronic HCV) can also be used.
- **Magnetic resonance imaging (MRI)** also detects macrostructural morphological changes (nodules, fissures, etc.), parenchymal changes (septa and fibrous bridges, regeneration nodules) and portal hypertension changes (splenomegaly, portosystemic varices, ascites and inter-asa oedema). The administration of IV contrast improves the visibility of cirrhotic changes and to differentiate from other vascular lesions such as portal arterial shunts or HCC (hepatocellular carcinoma).

Serum markers are non-specific and may be elevated in inflammation of other tissues, and some markers are secreted molecules such as bilirubin, alpha-fetoprotein (AFP), alpha-2-macroglobulin, haptoglobin and apolipoprotein A1. Individual serum biomarkers are not adequate for the diagnosis of liver cirrhosis, therefore biomarker panels have been developed for diagnostic use such as the

FIB-4 index, NFS, FibroTest, Forns index, Hepascore and Fibrometer and are frequently used in NASH patients (40) (42).

2.1.5.2. CHILD-PUGH, MELD and MELDNa SCALE

The **Child-Pugh scale** is a scale created to classify and evaluate the prognosis of mortality in cirrhotic patients. It was originally developed by Child and Turcotte in 1964 to select those patients who were candidates for elective surgery for portal decompression. This scale classifies patients with cirrhosis into three lettered categories: **A** (preserved liver function), **B** (significant compromise of liver function) and **C** (end-stage liver function). Initially this system was developed with five clinical and laboratory criteria: serum bilirubin, serum albumin, ascites, encephalopathy and clinical nutritional status. Years later, this scale was modified by Pugh, replacing clinical nutritional status with prothrombin time or INR, and renamed the Child-Pugh scale or modified Child-Pugh scale. It should be remembered that there are some limitations to The presence of subjective criteria (encephalopathy and ascites) and the omission of renal function (43).According to the sum of the points, the degree of chronic liver disease and the survival at one and two years are obtained:

Table 3. Child-Pugh scale

Parameters		Points allocated		
		1	2	3
Ascites		Absent	Slight	Moderate
Bilirubin, mg/dl		</= 2	2 Mar	> 3
Albumin, g/dl		> 3,5	2,8 - 3,5	< 2,8
Prothrombin time (seconds over control) / INR		1 - 3 s / INR <1,8	4 - 6 s / INR 1,8 - 2,3	>6 / INR >2,3
Encephalopathy (West-Haven)		No	Grade I - II	Grade III - IV
Grade	Points	Survival at one year(%)	Survival at 2 years (%)	
A: Disease well compensated	5 - 6	100	85	
B: Significant functional compromise	7 - 9	80	60	
C: Decompensated disease	10 - 15	45	35	

The MELD scale evaluates more objective and standardised parameters such as routine laboratory data (INR, bilirubin and creatinine), being a more accurate scale compared to Child-Pugh, with values between 6 (best prognosis) and 40 (worst prognosis) points. It is mostly used in the USA to reduce mortality in patients on the waiting list for a liver transplant. After several years, it was decided to modify and improve the MELD prediction value, implementing the serum sodium value **(MELD-Na)**, which provides greater accuracy in predicting mortality in patients on the transplant waiting list (44). Both scales are considered methods of prioritisation for transplantation and as prognostic for survival and mortality in cirrhotic patients. But as with any scale, it also has limitations in certain populations such as patients with sarcopenia and women with lower muscle mass, which reflect lower serum creatinine levels, leading to inaccurate values of their renal function, and it does not consider the aetiology of liver cirrhosis and does not predict risk in patients with ACLF (44) (45) .

2.2. DEFINITION OF HYPONATRAEMIA AND CLINICAL MANIFESTATIONS OF HYPONATRAEMIA

Hyponatraemia is an electrolyte disorder frequently observed in hospitalised patients, defined as a serum sodium concentration of less than 135 mEq/L (46) .

It is considered a subclinical entity, being of insidious onset, because the CNS has the ability to adapt to the hyponatraemic change in ECL by a compensatory reduction of intracellular osmolarity. Usually these types of patients are asymptomatic with serum sodium levels above 125 mEq/L, but certain symptoms such as headache, anorexia/hyporexia, asthenia, nausea, vomiting and alterations of the musculoskeletal system (sarcopenia, dynapenia, muscle spasms or fasciculations) may occur.

At levels below 120 mEq/L there is evidence of very serious complications such as: sensory impairment (stupor, obtundation or coma), tonic-clonic seizures, cardiac arrhythmias, cerebral oedema and hepatic encephalopathy, and death. Hyponatraemia has been shown to be an independent predictor of severity, longer hospital stay or ICU admission, increased risk of sepsis, and mortality, and the severity of clinical symptoms due to hyponatraemia correlates with osmolality and serum sodium level in extracellular fluid (47) (48).

2.3.HYPONATRAEMIA IN LIVER CIRRHOSIS

Hyponatraemia can be classified according to total free water, severity of symptoms, serum sodium and duration. According to total free water hyponatraemia is divided into hypovolaemic, normovolaemic and hypervolaemic or dilutional hyponatraemia. Hypervolaemic hyponatraemia occurs in 90% of patients with liver cirrhosis and is characterised by water loss to the third space (ascites, anasarca and lower limb oedema) due to hypersecretion of vasopressin and renal reabsorption of sodium and inability to excrete free water, whereas hypovolaemic hyponatraemia is caused by excessive use of diuretics or diarrhoea. Normovolaemic hyponatraemia is very rare in the setting of liver cirrhosis and is not widely described in the literature (48) (49).

Hyponatraemia can be classified according to its clinical severity as mild (few or no symptoms), moderate (nausea, confusion, headache, etc.) and severe or profound (vomiting, cardio respiratory collapse, convulsions and coma), and the same classification can be used but in the context of serum sodium values, being mild hyponatraemia with a serum sodium of 130-135 mmol/L, moderate with 125-129 mmol/L and severe with a natraemia <120 mmol/L (47).

Liver cirrhosis may present with hypervolaemic (the most common presentation) or hypovolaemic hyponatraemia, so urinary osmolality and fractional excretion of sodium (FENa) are considered to establish a more accurate diagnosis (48):

- **Urinary osmolality:** <150 mOsm/kg in hypovolaemic hyponatraemia due to diuretic use and >150 mOsm/kg in hypervolaemic hyponatraemia due to impaired free water excretion due to vasopressin.
- **FeNa:** In patients with normal renal function and hyponatraemia FeNa is 0.1%, while in hypovolaemic hyponatraemia it is <0.1% and >0.1% in hypervolaemic hyponatraemia.

Hyponatraemia is usually a late complication of liver cirrhosis, even being detected in Child A cirrhosis, but the neurological symptomatology of hyponatraemia cannot be related only to this water-electrolyte disruption, because the neurological symptoms (altered sensorium, fatigue, nausea and dizziness, gait instability and muscle cramps) may mimic hepatic encephalopathy or precipitate an episode of hepatic encephalopathy (48). Hyponatraemia can be defined in two distinct clinical settings: hyponatraemia in compensated cirrhosis and hyponatraemia in decompensated cirrhosis, which in turn is subdivided into hyponatraemia with neurological complications, hyponatraemia in refractory ascites and hyponatraemia in acute renal failure. Each clinical situation of hyponatraemia in liver cirrhosis is briefly explained below (48) (50) (51) (52) (53):

1. Hyponatraemia in compensated cirrhosis: Hyponatraemia does not usually occur in compensated cirrhosis and should be suspected only if there is exaggerated use of laxatives (hypovolaemic hyponatraemia) or normovolaemic hyponatraemia (hypothyroidism and adrenal insufficiency).

2. Hyponatraemia in decompensated cirrhosis:

● **Hyponatraemia with neurological complications:** Hyponatraemia in liver cirrhosis influences the occurrence of cerebral oedema, hyperammonaemia and increases the risk of developing hepatic encephalopathy due to adaptation to a hyponatraemic environment, oxidative stress and pro-inflammatory cytokine action.

● **Hyponatraemia in liver cirrhosis and refractory ascites**: Refractory ascites is defined as grade 3 ascites, treated with repeated evacuating paracentesis, adequate diuretic treatment and strict dietary sodium restriction. This refractory ascites is caused by prolonged hyperactivation of the RAAS, ADH and SNS leading to sodium and water retention, together with decreased oncotic pressure due to hypoalbuminaemia, increased interstitial capillary permeability and renal reduction/failure.

● **Hyponatraemia in acute renal failure and liver cirrhosis:** Acute renal failure in cirrhotics is caused by persistent renal hypoperfusion secondary to splanchnic vasodilatation, in addition to other related factors such as spontaneous bacterial peritonitis, infections, gastrointestinal bleeding and use of nephrotoxic drugs, and if renal damage persists; it could trigger a hepatorenal syndrome.

2.3.1. PATHOPHYSIOLOGY OF HYPONATRAEMIA IN LIVER CIRRHOSIS

The pathophysiology of hyponatraemia in liver cirrhosis is complex and involves a large number of pathophysiological mechanisms, but can be summarised in two major mechanisms (48) (54):

1. Splanchnic vasodilatation: Portal hypertension develops due to increased intravascular hepatic resistance and portal hyperflow, resulting in splanchnic vasodilatation due to the action of endogenous vasodilators (such as nitric oxide) and extrahepatic hyporereactivity to vasoconstrictors (e.g., thromboxane A2, angiotensin II, ADH, etc.); producing a reduction in effective arterial blood volume and renal perfusion, activating the renin-angiotensin-aldosterone system. thromboxane A2, angiotensin II, ADH, etc); producing a reduction in effective arterial blood volume and renal perfusion, activating the renin-angiotensin-aldosterone system (RAAS) and the Sympathetic Nervous System (SNS); the end result being sodium and water retention, ascites, lower limb oedema and dilutional hyponatraemia.

2. Osmotic and non-osmotic stimulation of vasopressin (ADH) secretion: While in a patient without pathology osmotic stimuli take priority, in the cirrhotic patient mainly non-osmotic factors, such as hypovolaemia or low effective arterial blood volume, are present due to nitric oxide-mediated splanchnic vasodilatation, and osmotic factors (hyponatraemia), leading to baroreceptor activation, ADH binding at vasopressin receptors (V2) and transport of aquaporins (AQP-2), which induce excessive tubular reabsorption of free water from the arteries. solutes in the collecting tubules, and dilutional hyponatraemia develops over a prolonged period of time.

2.4. TREATMENT OF HYPONATRAEMIA IN LIVER CIRRHOSIS

Treatment of hyponatraemia in cirrhotic patients varies depending on the clinical stage of the disease. As is well known, hyponatraemia in liver cirrhosis is a chronic and adaptive process, so patients may present asymptomatic or with symptoms similar to hepatic encephalopathy. It is not recommended to treat all cirrhotic patients with hyponatraemia because of the risk of pontine demyelination syndrome due to abrupt correction of serum sodium, and it is suggested to start treatment with a serum sodium value of less than 120 mmol/L and/or hyponatraemia with neurological symptoms.

The therapeutic conduct to be followed in patients with hypovolaemic hyponatraemia is based on the balanced use of crystalloids (sodium chloride 0.9% with correction of bicarbonate deficit) and anti-hyperkalemic measures (normosodic diet, 10% calcium gluconate or calcium chloride, glucose and insulin, salbutamol and loop and thiazide diuretics), while in asymptomatic patients with hypervolaemic hyponatraemia the following guidelines should be followed (47) (48) (49) (55) (56):

• **Discontinuation of diuretics and beta-blockers:** Diuretic use is an important pillar within the therapeutics of liver cirrhosis, and an aldosterone antagonist diuretic (spironolactone) and a loop diuretic (furosemide) are generally used in case of ascites; but bearing in mind that their chronic use produces hyponatraemia. Withdrawal of the diuretic should be controlled, due to the adverse effect of worsening ascites and limb oedema.

Beta-blockers are used in patients with liver cirrhosis as primary or secondary prophylaxis for variceal upper gastrointestinal bleeding, and should be discontinued if the mean arterial pressure (MAP) is <82 mmHg, because of the possibility of worsening ascites, hyponatraemia and increased mortality.

• **Fluid restriction:** It is advised to decrease fluid intake <750-500 ml in patients with natraemia <120 mmol/L until a negative water balance is achieved, but if patient tolerance is poor, a water restriction of 1 - 1.5 L, and discontinuation of sodium correction once the target natraemia (135-145 mmol/L) is reached.

• **Normotensive therapy:** Midodrine (antihypotensive) and octreotide (salvage therapy in irascible gastrointestinal bleeding) have been used in patients with persistent hypotension after discontinuation of beta-blockers and diuretics, and have been shown to improve MAP and treat hyponatraemia, especially in patients with hepatorenal syndrome, improving renal function considerably.

• **Correction of hyponatraemia deficit and hypokalaemia:** Correction of hyponatraemia should be carried out with extreme caution, avoiding a very accelerated correction that could lead to a pontine demyelination syndrome. Hypokalaemia caused by heavy use of diuretics and laxatives should also be corrected. Correction of this electrolyte has two advantages: it prevents the development of metabolic alkalosis (which can precipitate or aggravate hepatic encephalopathy by increasing renal glutaminase) and contributes to the correction of hyponatraemia, by electrolyte exchange with sodium,

Patients with severe and/or symptomatic hypervolaemic hyponatraemia require stricter therapeutic management and close monitoring, and in addition to the measures described above, the following are advised (48) (57) (58) (59):

• **20% albumin infusion:** Although the mechanism of action is not fully elucidated, it is thought that intravenous albumin increases renal perfusion due to its oncotic (VSAE) and non-oncotic (reduced RAAS action) properties. The recommended dose is 1 g/kg/h (maximum 100 g) and has been shown to be effective in several studies, but the major disadvantage is its high economic cost and difficult to acquire in developing and/or low-income countries.

More studies are needed to consider it as a treatment for hyponatraemia in liver cirrhosis, but it has shown efficacy in other pathologies such as: spontaneous bacterial peritonitis (SBP), hepatic encephalopathy, cirrhotic cardiomyopathy, hepatorenal syndrome and prophylaxis of post-paracentesis circulatory damage in large volume ascites.

• **Hypertonic 3% sodium chloride infusion:** The use of hypertonic saline should be reserved exclusively for patients with hyponatremia. <110 mmol/L and with neurological symptoms such as seizures, cardiopulmonary distress and altered sensorium. It is recommended to use boluses of 100 ml over 15-20 minutes, with a continuous maintenance infusion of 15-30 ml/hour, with a target increase of 4-6 mmol/L of serum sodium (maximum 9 mmol/L).

Desmopressin (synthetic analogue of antidiuretic hormone) can be added as a preventive measure for a pontine demyelination syndrome, in doses of 1-2 mcg c/6-8h for 24-48 hours until the target serum sodium level is reached. Another consideration is the deleterious effect of producing hypervolaemia in the hypertonic solution infusion, so loop diuretics may be added.

• **Use of vasopressin receptor antagonists (vaptans):** Vaptans are drugs that block the action of ADH at vasopressin receptors (V1 and V2) at the level of the renal collecting tubule, promoting free water excretion and increasing serum sodium. The most commonly used vaptans are conivaptan (IV only) and tolvaptan (oral), with tolvaptan being the most accessible; while chronic use of conivaptan has been shown to produce hypotension and recurrence of variceal bleeding in cirrhotic patients.

Prospective studies such as SALT (Study of Ascending Levels of Tolvaptan) and SALTWATER (Safety and sodium Assessment of Long-term Tovalptan With Hyponatremia) have demonstrated the efficacy of vaptans in the treatment of hyponatremia in cirrhotic patients, but it should be noted that the studies had certain limitations such as the focus on Syndrome of Inadequate Antidiuretic Hormone Secretion (SIADH) and a small group of cirrhotic patients in the studies. The most commonly reported adverse effects of tolvaptan use are oral xerostomia, polyuria, excessive daytime urination, thirst, fatigue and altered transaminases, which pose a potential risk in patients awaiting liver transplantation or with hepatorenal syndrome, but the FDA has not yet approved its use as a treatment for liver cirrhosis, except in clinical trials.

CHAPTER III

METHODOLOGY AND ANALYSIS OF RESULTS

3.1. RESEARCH DESIGN

An observational, retrospective, descriptive and cross-sectional study was carried out for this study.

3.2. STUDY POPULATION

3.2.1. UNIVERSE

All patients diagnosed with liver cirrhosis at the Hospital General del Norte de Guayaquil Ceibos during the time period from January 2021 to June 2022, with a total of 316 patients.

3.2.2. SAMPLE

From the total universe of 316 patients, the following inclusion criteria were applied, resulting in a sample of 111 patients.

3.2.2.1. INCLUSION CRITERIA

A. Patients with an established diagnosis of liver cirrhosis (ICD-10: K74) and hyponatraemia according to laboratory data.

B. Patients with complete medical history and complete laboratory tests.
C. Patients admitted to the Gastroenterology area of the Hospital General Norte de Guayaquil IESS Los Ceibos in the period of time to be studied (January 2021 - June 2022).

3.2.2.2 EXCLUSION CRITERIA

A. Patients with unreported or incomplete laboratory results.
B. Patients differential diagnosis of cirrhosis (heart failure).(heart failure).

C. Patients with a request for voluntary medical discharge.

3.3. COMPUTERISED DATA COLLECTION AND MANAGEMENT

The data used in this study were collected through the review of medical records in the AS400 system of patients hospitalised with a diagnosis of liver cirrhosis at the Hospital General del Norte de Guayaquil IESS Los Ceibos during the period from January 2021 to June 2022 in the hospitalisation unit of Gastroenterology (Gastroenterology - HO), in which a database was created in Microsoft Excel 2016, including all the variables to be used in the study. In addition, online calculators were used to obtain the Child-Pugh scale scores on the website: Rapid Critical Care Consult (https://www.rccc.eu/).

3.4. STATISTICAL ANALYSIS

All data were collected in SPSS v.25 software and Excel 2016 for tabulation and subsequent analysis, in addition to the preparation of tables and graphs. For the descriptive analysis, numerical variables were averaged by standard deviation, while frequencies and percentages were calculated for non-numerical variables. Chi-square was used for the numerical variables, and p-values <0.05 were considered statistically significant.

3.5. RESULTS

For the development of this research, the Statistics Department of the Hospital General del Norte de Guayaquil IESS Los Ceibos provided us, through the indicated communication channels, with a database of patients with cirrhosis and hyponatremia hospitalised in the period from **January 2021 to June 2022.** The study included a universe of 316 patients, of which 120 patients were identified as meeting the inclusion criteria for hospitalisation in the Gastroenterology area of the Hospital IESS Los Ceibos and 9 patients were excluded, resulting in a total of 111 patients **(Figure 4)** with cirrhosis and hyponatraemia **(Figure 4).**Regarding the characteristics of the patients according to their sex, age, drugs and hospital stay **(Table 4)**; it is recognised that 50.5% are women, while the remaining 49.5% belong to the male sex **(Graph 5).** In terms of age, the predominant age range was 51 to 70 years with 64.9%, followed by 30.6% for those aged 71 to 91 years; it was also recognised that 63.1% use drugs (diuretics) **(Figure 6).** On the other hand, 72.1% had a hospital stay of 1 to 15 days, while 22.5% were hospitalised for 16 to 30 days **(Figure 7).**To estimate the prevalence of degrees of hyponatraemia in patients with liver cirrhosis), the following formula was considered to identify the prevalence:Prevalence = New and pre-existing cases in a period * 100 Total population in periodWithin the Hospital General del Norte de Guayaquil IESS Los Ceibos, a total of 111 cases of cirrhotic patients with hyponatraemia were identified during the period January 2021 to June 2022. During this same period, the number of patients with liver cirrhosis seen in the hospital was 316 patients; considering the previously established formula, the overall prevalence of hyponatraemia in patients with cirrhosis was determined to be 35.1%.With regard to the degrees of hyponatraemia, there is a higher prevalence of mild hyponatraemia with 23.7%, moderate hyponatraemia with a prevalence of 10.1% and severe hyponatraemia with a prevalence of 1.3% **(Table 5)**. In summary, the prevalence of hyponatremiavaries; however, the most common degrees are mild and moderate compared to severe hyponatraemia **(Figure 8)**.

Regarding the relationship of the degree of hyponatraemia with the comorbidities associated with liver cirrhosis, the variables were crossed using a Chi-square test and it was identified that only cancer was related to the degrees of hyponatraemia, obtaining a p-value of 0.049 (less than 0.05) **(Table 6).** In this setting, the presence of cancer leads to a moderate degree of hyponatraemia. In contrast, comorbidities such as hypertension, diabetes mellitus, chronic kidney disease and tuberculosis (TB) were not significantly related to the degrees of hyponatraemia with a significance greater than 0.05 (Figure 9). **(Figure 9).**

A correlation of the severity of cirrhosis according to the Child-Pugh scale and the degree of hyponatraemia of the patients studied was performed, and under a descriptive approach, it was determined that 31.5% of cirrhotic patients with a mild degree of hyponatraemia presented a level B severity (moderate liver disease) of cirrhosis. This means that the patient with a class A cirrhosis with compromised liver function and a better prognosis, whereas, 22.5% exhibited a level C indicating severe cirrhosis with very impaired liver function and a poorer prognosis **(Table 7)**. It is worth mentioning that a relationship between the two variables was not identified by observing a p-value greater than 0.05 (0.256) in the Chi-Square test **(Figure 10)**.In identifying the stage of cirrhosis in which the different degrees of hyponatraemia occur most frequently in the population studied, it was recognised that 51.4% of cirrhotic patients with a mild degree of hyponatraemia had decompensated cirrhosis, while 16.2% had compensated cirrhosis **(Figure 11 and Table 8)**. It is worth mentioning that decompensated cirrhosis also predominated in the moderate and severe degrees of hyponatraemia with 26.1% and 2.7% respectively, recognising that during this phase the liver functionality is affected by chronic changes in its architecture and vascularity, precipitating portal hypertension and the onset of hyponatraemia. In the study, when determining the relationship between the degree of hyponatraemia and the most frequent complications in cirrhotic patients, it was found that 27% of cirrhotic patients with mild hyponatraemia had a grade 0 in the West Haven criteria, indicating the absence of hepatic encephalopathy. In contrast, 16.2% of patients with mild hyponatraemia had grade 2 encephalopathy according to the West Haven classification **(table 9).**

On the other hand, most patients with mild hyponatraemia (40.5%) presented oesophageal varices, although those with moderate hyponatraemia did not present this complication, while 38.7% with mild hyponatraemia presented ascites **(Figure 12).** With respect to severe hyponatraemia, only 3.6% reported non-variceal upper gastrointestinal haemorrhage (NAUH). Statistically, only HDA was related to the degree of hyponatraemia with a p-value of less than 0.05 (0.032) in the Chi-square test **(Table 9).**

For our prevalence study, cross-tabulations were performed to determine the correlation between the different variables to be studied. Considering the crosstabulation of the variables age and sex, it was identified that cirrhotic patients with hyponatraemia belong mainly to the female sex, with a predominance of patients aged 51 to 70 years (32.4%) **(graph 13).** This age range is equally prevalent in male patients with 32.4%; it is worth mentioning that a relationship between both criteria was not identified as a significance greater than 0.05 (0.909) was observed **(Table 10).**

With respect to the variables of age and sex with the degree of hyponatraemia, it was shown that 35.1% of female patients with liver cirrhosis have a mild degree of hyponatraemia, as do 32.4% of men; however, it is the latter who predominate in the level of moderate hyponatraemia **(Table 11).** In terms of age, the range with the highest number of cases of mild and moderate hyponatraemia was the aged 51 to 70 years (64.9%); no correlation between the variables was identified with a p-value greater than 0.005 **(Figure 14).**

Regarding sex and age with the clinical stage of liver cirrhosis (compensated or decompensated), it was found that cirrhotic patients with a decompensated state are mostly men (41.4%); however, in compensated cirrhosis, women predominate with 11.7% **(Table 12).** Similarly, people between 51 and 70 years of age stand out for maintaining a decompensated clinical stage (55%); statistically, age was related to the clinical stages of cirrhosis by obtaining a p-value of less than 0.05 (0.002) **(Figure 15).**When relating sex to the complications of liver cirrhosis (hepatic encephalopathy, oesophageal varices, upper gastrointestinal bleeding, jaundice and ascites) it was found that 19.8% of cirrhotic patients with hyponatraemia had no hepatic encephalopathy, while 16.2% who were identified as having grade 2 hepatic encephalopathy were men **(Table 13) (Figure 16).** Oesophageal varices predominated in females with 33.3%, while cases of ascites occurred mostly in males with 29.7%. On the other hand, it was observed that oesophageal varices were related to sex, with a significance of less than 0.05 (0.046) **(Table 13).**

Regarding age and complications of liver cirrhosis, it was observed that the majority of patients with grade 0 West Haven criteria for hepatic encephalopathy were between 51 and 70 years of age (20.7%), with oesophageal varices (36%), ADH (23.4%) and ascites (38.7%) **(Table 14) (Figure 17).** No relationship between complications of liver cirrhosis and age was observed given a p-value greater than 0

3.6. DISCUSSION

Hyponatraemia is a medical condition characterised by low serum sodium levels that presents as a disruption of the osmotic balance in the body as a result of increased free water due to difficulties in its excretion (60).

The literature establishes that, in patients with cirrhosis, hyponatraemia occurs when serum sodium is 130 mEq/L. Its clinical manifestations can range from subtle symptoms, such as nausea and confusion, to severe complications, such as cerebral oedema and seizures (48).

It is essential to recognise that hyponatraemia in patients with liver cirrhosis represents a significant healthcare challenge, as the presence of hyponatraemia in this setting has been shown to be associated with increased morbidity and mortality (61).

Consequently, the main objective of this study was to estimate the prevalence of the degree of hyponatraemia in patients with liver cirrhosis admitted to the Gastroenterology Department at the Hospital General del Norte de Guayaquil IESS Los Ceibos in the period from January 2021 to June 2022. The results showed that cirrhotic patients with hyponatraemia are mostly women, predominantly aged 51 to 91 years; in addition, it was identified that a large proportion of patients had a hospital stay of 1 to 15 days, and used drugs (diuretics). Regarding demographic criteria, the study by Younes et al (2021) identified that hyponatraemia was present in 36.9% of patients with cirrhosis, where 53.12% were male and 46.8% female, which differs from current findings (61). However, the mean age was 53.7 ± 11.3 years. Likewise, in the research by Defás and Mogro (2021) there was a predominance of male (56.57%) over female (43.43%), while the mean age was 65 years. Regarding hospital stay, the patients with hyponatraemia lasted an average of 9.3 days, somewhat in line with the current results (62).Among the comorbidities associated with liver cirrhosis that the patients presented, arterial hypertension (57.7%), diabetes mellitus (46.8%), chronic kidney disease (19.8%), cancer (15.3%) and, to a lesser extent, tuberculosis (2.7%) stand out. These data are consistent with the findings of Defás and Mogro (2021) where the predominant comorbidities were hypertension (36.36%), diabetes (23.23%) and chronic kidney disease (9.6%) (62). In summary, these three diseases are found to be the most frequent comorbidities in cirrhotic patients with hyponatraemia due to the direct effects of liver disease on the cardiovascular system, glucose metabolism and renal function, which are aggravated by the presence of hyponatraemia.Mild hyponatraemia predominated in cases of arterial hypertension, diabetes mellitus and chronic kidney disease; however, moderate hyponatraemia predominated in cases of cancer and tuberculosis. It is worth mentioning that there is a limited number of cases of severe hyponatraemia, with a proportion of 3.6% (4 cases) identified in patients with diabetes and hypertension being attributed to this level. This compared to the mild and moderate levels, where the former held a share of 67.6% and the latter 28.8%. In contrast to the current findings, in the work of Younes et al (2021) moderate hyponatraemia was predominant with 21.5%, followed by mild (9.2%) and severe (6.2%) (61). Based on the results obtained and the literature reviewed, it is determined that mild hyponatraemia is the most common form due to factors such as excessive fluid intake and the use of diuretics, which result in a mild dilution of blood sodium levels, while severe hyponatracmia is the least common.In terms of the severity of cirrhosis, a predominance of level B severity was observed, with cases of mild hyponatraemia standing out. In second place, level C severity was found, followed by level A, both with a higher number of cases of mild hyponatraemia. which refers to mild hyponatraemia. In the work of Defás and Mogro (2021) it was observed that of the patients with hyponatraemia, 62.04% had a level B severity of cirrhosis, 39.37% a grade A and 75% a level C (62) . Whereas, in the study by Pradeep and Sindhura (2022) 76.6% had a B/C level and 50% an A level, which is consistent with the current results (63). This allows us to recognise that the majority of patients maintain a moderately compromised liver function, with a higher risk of complications and a lower survival compared to level A.On the other hand, most of the patients were in the decompensated cirrhosis stage, while only 22 cases showed a compensated stage of cirrhosis, in both cases, the degree of mild hyponatraemia was notable. In the study by Pradeep and Sindhura (2022) it was observed that patients with decompensated cirrhosis exhibit different complications that are associated with higher mortality in hospitalised patients such as ascites, hepatic encephalopathy and upper gastrointestinal haemorrhage and even Parkinson's disease, increasing morbidity and mortality in patients (63). Regarding complications, the majority of patients reported a grade 0 on the West Haven criteria (33.3%), indicating the absence of hepatic encephalopathy; however, 27.9% reported a grade 2 and 22.5% reported a grade 1. In smaller proportions, cases of non-variceal upper gastrointestinal haemorrhage (NAUH) and jaundice were reported, with a predominance of mild hyponatraemia. In the work of Defás and Mogro (2021) the predominant complications were oesophageal varices (51.52%), ascites (53.03%), variceal bleeding (34.85%), hepatic encephalopathy (28.28%), hepatorenal syndrome (HRS) (30.81%) and jaundice (15.66%) (62). Similarly, in the study by Bhandari and Chaudhary (2021) the predominant complications were oedema (100%), ascites (93.6%), pallor (93.6%), upper gastrointestinal bleeding (74.5%), jaundice (72.3%), hepatic hepatic encephalopathy (46.8%), among others (64). Meanwhile, Pradeep and Sindhura (2022) noted that patients with hyponatraemia had ascites (74.4%) and hepatic encephalopathy (85.4%) (63).The results associated with hepatic encephalopathy are consistent with the findings of Younes et al (2021), since, in their work 32.3% had no hepatic encephalopathy, while in our study 20.8% indicated grade 1, 23.8% grade 2, 12.3% grade 3 and 10.8% grade 4 (61). This shows that hyponatraemia tends to affect brain function in cirrhotic patients, predisposing them to exposure to hepatic encephalopathy.According to Younes et al (2021), the risk of developing these complications is directly proportional to the degree of hyponatraemia, stating that several studies have shown that severe hyponatraemia is associated with a higher severity of hepatic encephalopathy (61). However, in the current study, this premise is not corroborated by showing a p-value > 0.05 and highlighting that the 4 cases of severe hyponatraemia occurred in patients with grade 1 and 2 hepatic encephalopathy. The overall prevalence of hyponatraemia in cirrhotic patients was 35.1%; however, by degree of hyponatraemia, mild hyponatraemia stands out with 23.7%, followed by moderate with 10.1% and severe with 1.3%. In the work of Attar (2019), the prevalence of hyponatraemia in patients with cirrhosis was identified as 22% (47), with severe hyponatraemia having a prevalence of 6%; while in the study by Ordoñez and Yperti (2023), the prevalence rate of severe hyponatraemia was 6.2%, with a greater predominance in women (65). On the other hand, in the study by Bhandari and Chaudhary (2021) the prevalence of hyponatraemia was 41.22% being higher in males (64). In the study by Pradeep and Sindhura (2022) the overall prevalence of hyponatraemia was 75% (63); while Bashir et al (2019) in their study highlights a prevalence of 47.9% (66). According to Defás and Mogro (2021) hyponatraemia is prevalent in 20-50% of cirrhotic patients and is relatively high (66). During the study there were certain limitations, such as the exclusion of patients due to lack of information or who had an ICD-10 diagnosis that did not correspond to the inclusion criteria; in addition to the fact that in some patients the specific aetiology of liver cirrhosis was not identified, due to incomplete anamnesis, the absence of complementary studies (due to lack of reagents or omission of laboratory results) or other complementary studies were not reported in the clinical history by omission or the patient performed the studies in a particular way, or a late hospitalisation with decompensated cirrhosis and recent diagnosis, which could lead to an underestimation of our results.

CHAPTER IV
CONCLUSIONS AND RECOMMENDATIONS

4.1. CONCLUSIONS

1. The prevalence of hyponatraemia in patients with cirrhosis overall was 35.1%, with a predominance of mild hyponatraemia with a prevalence of 67.6%, moderate hyponatraemia with 28.8% and severe hyponatraemia with 3.6%.

2. Cancer was the only comorbidity identified as being related to degrees of hyponatraemia (p-value of $0.049 < 0.05$). 8.1% had moderate hyponatraemia.

3. No relationship was identified between severity of cirrhosis and degree of hyponatraemia (p-value $0.256 > 0.05$); however, a predominance of Child-Pugh B (42.3%) was recognised, where 31.5% had mild hyponatraemia.

4. The stage of decompensated cirrhosis is where most cases were identified (80.2%), with 51.4% having mild hyponatraemia, 26.1% moderate hyponatraemia and 2.7% severe hyponatraemia.

5. Non-variceal upper gastrointestinal bleeding (NAUH) was the only complication related to the degree of hyponatraemia (p-value $0.032 < 0.05$) in our study, with 23.4% with mild hyponatraemia, 10.8% with moderate hyponatraemia and 3.6% with severe hyponatraemia.

4.2. RECOMMENDATIONS

1. It is suggested to the scientific community to carry out new studies on the prevalence of hyponatraemia in cirrhotic patients in the various health centres in the country due to the lack of data in this line of research.

2. Due to the association between cancer and hyponatraemia levels, continuous monitoring of sodium levels in cancer patients is recommended, which could improve quality of life and reduce morbidity and mortality.

3. Apply methods of early detection of decompensation in cirrhotic patients with comorbidities to avoid the development of a higher degree of hyponatraemia leading to short and long term complications.

4. The institution is recommended to develop educational programmes aimed at patients with cirrhosis to explain the importance of complying with medical recommendations and to prevent the development of complications.

5. Implement a long-term follow-up protocol for patients with liver cirrhosis and hyponatraemia for early detection of complications and improved survival.

REFERENCES

1. Poveda KAF, Arias JEM, Subia DLF, Castro AMM. Liver cirrhosis: epidemiological profile and quality of life. Teodoro Maldonado Carbo Hospital. Period 2014
- 2015. Digital Science [Internet]. October 4, 2019 [cited 2023 July 3];3(4):82-100.Available from:
https://cienciadigital.org/revistacienciadigital2/index.php/CienciaDigital/article/view/ 936
2. IHME. Institute for Health Metrics and Evaluation. 2020 [cited 3 July 2023]. Cirrhosis and other chronic liver diseases due to other causes - Level 4 cause. Available from:
https://www.healthdata.org/results/gbd_summaries/2019/cirrhosis-and-other-chronic- liver-diseases-due-to-other-causes-level-4-cause
3. American College of Gastroenterology [Internet]. 2012 [cited 3 July 2023]. Liver Cirrhosis. Available from: https://gi.org/topics/liver-cirrhosis/
4. INEC. Vital Statistics. Registro Estadístico de Defunciones Generales de 2021 - Buscar con Google [Internet]. 2022 [cited 3 July 2023]. Available from: https://www.ecuadorencifras.gob.ec/documentos/web-inec/Poblacion_y_Demografia/Defunciones_General_2021/Principales_resultados_ EDG_2021_v2.pdf.
5. Bernal JFM, Morales EL, Sandino NJ, Franco DM. Liver cirrhosis or chronic acute liver failure: definition and classification. Revista Repertorio de Medicina y Cirugía [Internet]. July 14, 2022 [cited July 3, 2023];31(2):112-22. Available from: https://revistas.fucsalud.edu.co/index.php/repertorio/article/view/1052
6. Smith A, Baumgartner K, Bositis C. Cirrhosis: Diagnosis and Management. afp [Internet]. December 15, 2019 [cited July 3, 2023];100(12):759-70. Available from: https://www.aafp.org/pubs/afp/issues/2019/1215/p759.html
7. Mellado-Orellana R, Sánchez-Herrera D, Deschamps-Corona A, Núñez-Hernández JC, Díaz-Greene EJ, Rodríguez-Weber FL. Hyponatraemia for beginners. Med Int Mex [Internet]. 2022 [cited 2022 Oct 26];38(2):397-408. Available from: https://www.medigraphic.com/cgi-bin/new/resumen.cgi?IDARTICULO=104967
8. Alukal JJ, John S, Thuluvath PJ. Hyponatremia in Cirrhosis: An Update. Official journal of the American College of Gastroenterology | ACG [Internet]. November 2020 [cited 2022 Oct 26];115(11):1775-85. Available from: https://journals.lww.com/ajg/Abstract/2020/11000/Hyponatremia_in_Cirrhosis An_ Update.11.aspx

9. Younas A, Riaz J, Chughtai T, Maqsood H, Saim M, Qazi S, et al. Hyponatremia and Its Correlation With Hepatic Encephalopathy and Severity of Liver Disease. Cureus. February 6, 2021;13(2):e13175.

10. Solís Alcívar DC, Bermúdez Garcell AJ, Serrano Gámez NB, Teruel Ginés R, Castro Maquilón AG, Solís Alcívar DC, et al. Effects of alcohol on the onset of liver cirrhosis. Correo Científico Médico [Internet]. June 2020 [cited 3 July 2023];24(2):743-63. Available from: http://scielo.sld.cu/scielo.php?script=sci_abstract&pid=S1560-43812020000200743&lng=en&nrm=iso&tlng=en

11. PAHO/WHO. Hepatitis [Internet]. 2019 [cited 3 July 2023]. Available from: https://www.paho.org/es/temas/hepatitis

12. Corrales Alonso S, Hernández Hernández R, González Báez A, Vanterpool Héctor M, Rangel Lorenzo E, Villar Ortiz D, et al. Descriptive study of patients with liver cirrhosis of viral etiology in the province of Matanzas. Revista Médica Electrónica [Internet]. April 2021 [cited 3 July 2023];43(2):3074-90. Available from: http://scielo.sld.cu/scielo.php?script=sci_abstract&pid=S1684-18242021000203074&lng=en&nrm=iso&tlng=en

13. Ospino Rodriguez M, Licona Vera E, Raad Sarabia M, Betancur Vásquez C, Gómez Álvarez L. Non-alcoholic steatohepatitis: From pathophysiology to diagnosis. Archives of Medicine [Internet]. 2022 [cited 2023 July 3];18(8):2. Available from: https://dialnet.unirioja.es/servlet/articulo?codigo=8693570

14. Vera Mesias MM, Parrales Carvajal JM, Rodríguez Parrales DH. Autoimmune hepatitis, clinical forms, diagnosis and prognosis. Polo del Conocimiento: Revista científico - profesional [Internet]. 2021 [cited July 3, 2023];6(7):61-77. Available at: https://dialnet.unirioja.es/servlet/articulo?codigo=8017035

15. Weersink RA, Burger DM, Hayward KL, Taxis K, Drenth JPH, Borgsteede SD. Safe use of medication in patients with cirrhosis: pharmacokinetic and pharmacodynamic considerations. Expert Opinion on Drug Metabolism & Toxicology [Internet]. January 2, 2020 [cited July 3, 2023];16(1):45-57. Available from: https://doi.org/10.1080/17425255.2020.1702022

16. Sandhu N, Navarro V. Drug-Induced Liver Injury in GI Practice. Hepatology Communications [Internet]. 2020 [cited 2023 July 3];4(5):631-45. Available from: https://onlinelibrary.wiley.com/doi/abs/10.1002/hep4.1503

17. Parola M, Pinzani M. Liver fibrosis: Pathophysiology, pathogenetic targets and clinical issues. Molecular Aspects of Medicine [Internet]. February 2019 [cited 2023 July 3];65:37-55. Available from: https://linkinghub.elsevier.com/retrieve/pii/S0098299718300700

18. Roehlen N, Crouchet E, Baumert TF. Liver Fibrosis: Mechanistic Concepts and Therapeutic Perspectives. Cells [Internet]. April 2020 [cited 2022 Oct 26];9(4):875. Available from: https://www.mdpi.com/2073-4409/9/4/875

19. Gunarathne LS, Rajapaksha H, Shackel N, Angus PW, Herath CB. Cirrhotic portal hypertension: From pathophysiology to novel therapeutics. World J Gastroenterol [Internet]. October 28, 2020 [cited July 3, 2023];26(40):6111-40. Available from: https://www.ncbi.nlm.nih.gov/pmc/articles/PMC7596642/

20. D'Amico G, Morabito A, D'Amico M, Pasta L, Malizia G, Rebora P, et al. New concepts on the clinical course and stratification of compensated and decompensated cirrhosis. Hepatol Int [Internet]. February 2018 [cited 3 July 2023];12(S1):34-43. Available from: http://link.springer.com/10.1007/s12072-017- 9808-z.

21. Sharma B, John S. Hepatic Cirrhosis. In: StatPearls [Internet]. Treasure Island (FL): StatPearls Publishing; 2023 [cited 2023 July 3]. Available from: http://www.ncbi.nlm.nih.gov/books/NBK482419/

22. Lesmana CRA, Raharjo M, Gani RA. Managing liver cirrhotic complications: Overview of esophageal and gastric varices. Clin Mol Hepatol [Internet]. Oct 1, 2020 [cited July 3, 2023];26(4):444-60. Available from: http://www.e- cmh.org/journal/view.php?doi=10.3350/cmh.2020.0022

23. Jakab SS, Garcia-Tsao G. SCREENING AND SURVEILLANCE OF VARICOSE VEINS IN PATIENTS WITH CIRRHOSIS. Clin Gastroenterol Hepatol [Internet]. January 2019 [cited July 3, 2023];17(1):26-9. Available from: https://www.ncbi.nlm.nih.gov/pmc/articles/PMC6139072/

24. Wilkins T, Wheeler B, Carpenter M. Upper Gastrointestinal Bleeding in Adults: Evaluation and Management. afp [Internet]. March 1, 2020 [cited July 3, 2023];101(5):294-300. Available from: https://www.aafp.org/pubs/afp/issues/2020/0301/p294.html

25. Custovic N, Husic-Selimovic A, Srsen N, Prohic D. Comparison of Glasgow- Blatchford Score and Rockall Score in Patients with Upper Gastrointestinal Bleeding. Med Arch [Internet]. August 2020 [cited 3 July 2023];74(4):270-4. Available from: https://www.ncbi.nlm.nih.gov/pmc/articles/PMC7520069/

26. Engelmann C, Clària J, Szabo G, Bosch J, Bernardi M. Pathophysiology of decompensated cirrhosis: Portal hypertension, circulatory dysfunction, inflammation, metabolism and mitochondrial dysfunction. Journal of Hepatology [Internet]. July 1, 2021 [cited 2022 Oct 26];75:S49-66. Available from: https://www.journal-of-hepatology.eu/article/S0168-8278(21)00002- 7/fulltext

27. Rudler M, Mallet M, Sultanik P, Bouzbib C, Thabut D. Optimal management of ascites. Liver International [Internet]. 2020 [cited 3 July 2023];40(S1):128-
35. Available at: https://onlinelibrary.wiley.com/doi/abs/10.1111/liv.14361

28. Garbuzenko DV, Arefyev NO. Current approaches to the management of patients with cirrhotic ascites. World J Gastroenterol [Internet]. July 28, 2019 [cited July 3, 2023];25(28):3738-52. Available from:
https://www.ncbi.nlm.nih.gov/pmc/articles/PMC6676543/

29. Joseph A, Samant H. Jaundice. In: StatPearls [Internet]. Treasure Island (FL): StatPearls Publishing; 2023 [cited 2023 July 3]. Available from: http://www.ncbi.nlm.nih.gov/books/NBK544252/

30. Pavlovic Markovic A, Stojkovic Lalosevic M, Mijac DD, Milovanovic T, Dragasevic S, Sokic Milutinovic A, et al. Jaundice as a Diagnostic and Therapeutic Problem: A General Practitioner's Approach. Digestive Diseases [Internet]. May 20, 2021 [cited July 3, 2023];40(3):362-9. Available from: https://doi.org/10.1159/000517301

31. Weissenborn K. Hepatic Encephalopathy: Definition, Clinical Grading and Diagnostic Principles. Drugs [Internet]. 2019 [cited 2023 July 3];79(Suppl 1):5-
9. Available from: https://www.ncbi.nlm.nih.gov/pmc/articles/PMC6416238/

32. Dellatore P, Cheung M, Mahpour NY, Tawadros A, Rustgi VK. Clinical Manifestations of Hepatic Encephalopathy. Clin Liver Dis. May 2020;24(2):189- 96.

33. Rose CF, Amodio P, Bajaj JS, Dhiman RK, Montagnese S, Taylor-Robinson SD, et al. Hepatic encephalopathy: Novel insights into classification, pathophysiology and therapy. J Hepatol. Dec 2020;73(6):1526-47.

34. Kabaria S, Dalal I, Gupta K, Bhurwal A, Minacapelli CD, Catalano C, et al. Hepatic Encephalopathy: A Review. EMJ [Internet]. August 5, 2021 [cited July 3, 2023];9(1):89-97. Available from:
https://www.emjreviews.com/hepatology/article/hepatic-encephalopathy-a-review/

35. Chen Z, Ruan J, Li D, Wang M, Han Z, Qiu W, et al. The Role of Intestinal Bacteria and Gut-Brain Axis in Hepatic Encephalopathy. Front Cell Infect Microbiol [Internet]. January 21, 2021 [cited July 3, 2023];10:595759. Available from: https://www.ncbi.nlm.nih.gov/pmc/articles/PMC7859631/

36. Leidi A, Pisaturo M, Fumeaux T. Malnutrition-related hyperammonemic encephalopathy presenting with burst suppression: a case report. Journal of Medical Case Reports [Internet]. August 10, 2019 [cited 2023 July 3];13(1):248. Available from: https://doi.org/10.1186/s13256-019-2185-6

37. Schindler P, Heinzow H, Trebicka J, Wildgruber M. Shunt-Induced Hepatic Encephalopathy in TIPS: Current Approaches and Clinical Challenges. J Clin Med [Internet]. November 23, 2020 [cited July 3, 2023];9(11):3784. Available from: https://www.ncbi.nlm.nih.gov/pmc/articles/PMC7700586/

38. Butterworth RF. Hepatic Encephalopathy in Cirrhosis: Pathology and Pathophysiology. Drugs [Internet]. 2019 [cited 2023 July 3];79(Suppl 1):17-21. Available at: https://www.ncbi.nlm.nih.gov/pmc/articles/PMC6416236/

39. Karanfilian BV, Cheung M, Dellatore P, Park T, Rustgi VK. Laboratory Abnormalities of Hepatic Encephalopathy. Clin Liver Dis. May 2020;24(2):197-208.

40. Lurie Y, Webb M, Cytter-Kuint R, Shteingart S, Lederkremer GZ. Non-invasive diagnosis of liver fibrosis and cirrhosis. World J Gastroenterol [Internet]. November 7, 2015 [cited July 3, 2023];21(41):11567-83. Available from: https://www.ncbi.nlm.nih.gov/pmc/articles/PMC4631961/

41. Gheorghe G, Bungău S, Ceobanu G, Ilie M, Bacalbaşa N, Bratu OG, et al. The non-invasive assessment of hepatic fibrosis. Journal of the Formosan Medical Association [Internet]. Feb. 1, 2021 [cited July 3, 2023];120(2):794-803. Available at: https://www.sciencedirect.com/science/article/pii/S0929664620303934

42. Campos-Murguía A, Ruiz-Margáin A, González-Regueiro JA, Macías-Rodríguez RU. Clinical assessment and management of liver fibrosis in non-alcoholic fatty liver disease. World J Gastroenterol [Internet]. Oct 21, 2020 [cited July 3, 2023];26(39):5919-43. Available from: https://www.ncbi.nlm.nih.gov/pmc/articles/PMC7584064/

43. Tsoris A, Marlar CA. Use Of The Child Pugh Score In Liver Disease. In: StatPearls [Internet]. Treasure Island (FL): StatPearls Publishing; 2023 [cited 2023 July 3]. Available from: http://www.ncbi.nlm.nih.gov/books/NBK542308/

44. Ruf A, Dirchwolf M, Freeman RB. From Child-Pugh to MELD score and beyond: Taking a walk down memory lane. Annals of Hepatology [Internet]. January 1, 2022 [cited July 3, 2023];27(1):100535. Available from. https://www.sciencedirect.com/science/article/pii/S1665268121002349

45. Trivedi HD. The Evolution of the MELD Score and Its Implications in Liver Transplant Allocation: A Beginner's Guide for Trainees. ACG Case Rep J [Internet]. May 4, 2022 [cited July 3, 2023];9(5):e00763. Available from: https://www.ncbi.nlm.nih.gov/pmc/articles/PMC9287268/

46. Mejía-Sandoval HJ, Castellanos-Bueno R, Rangel-Rivera DA, Rangel-Rivera KL, Mejía-Sandoval HJ, Castellanos-Bueno R, et al. Practical aspects for the classification, diagnosis and management of hyponatremia in the

hospitalized patient. Medicas UIS [Internet]. August 2020 [cited 3 July 2023];33(2):85-93. Available from: http://www.scielo.org.co/scielo.php?script=sci_abstract&pid=S0121-03192020000200010&lng=en&nrm=iso&tlng=en

47. Attar B. Approach to Hyponatremia in Cirrhosis. Clinical Liver Disease [Internet]. 2019 [cited 2022 Oct 26];13(4):98-101. Available from: https://onlinelibrary.wiley.com/doi/abs/10.1002/cld.790

48. Praharaj DL, Anand AC. Clinical Implications, Evaluation, and Management of Hyponatremia in Cirrhosis. J Clin Exp Hepatol [Internet]. 2022 [cited 2023 July 3];12(2):575-94. Available from: https://www.ncbi.nlm.nih.gov/pmc/articles/PMC9077240/

49. Baiges A, Hernández-Gea V. Management of Liver Decompensation in Advanced Chronic Liver Disease: Ascites, Hyponatremia, and Gastroesophageal Variceal Bleeding. Clin Drug Investig [Internet]. 2022 [cited 2023 July 3];42(Suppl 1):25-31. Available from: https://www.ncbi.nlm.nih.gov/pmc/articles/PMC9205794/

50. Rondon-Berrios H, Velez JCQ. Hyponatremia in Cirrhosis. Clin Liver Dis [Internet]. May 2022 [cited 2023 July 3];26(2):149-64. Available from: https://www.ncbi.nlm.nih.gov/pmc/articles/PMC9060324/

51. Chaney A. A Review for the Practicing Clinician: Hepatorenal Syndrome, a Form of Acute Kidney Injury, in Patients with Cirrhosis. Clinical and Experimental Gastroenterology [Internet]. December 31, 2021 [cited July 3, 2023];14:385-96. Available from: https://www.tandfonline.com/doi/abs/10.2147/CEG.S323778

52. Gupta K, Bhurwal A, Law C, Ventre S, Minacapelli CD, Kabaria S, et al. Acute kidney injury and hepatorenal syndrome in cirrhosis. World J Gastroenterol [Internet]. July 14, 2021 [cited July 3, 2023];27(26):3984-4003. Available from: https://www.ncbi.nlm.nih.gov/pmc/articles/PMC8311533/

53. Kulkarni AV, Kumar P, Sharma M, Sowmya TR, Talukdar R, Rao PN, et al. Pathophysiology and Prevention of Paracentesis-induced Circulatory Dysfunction: A Concise Review. J Clin Transl Hepatol [Internet]. March 28, 2020 [cited July 3, 2023];8(1):42-8. Available from: https://www.ncbi.nlm.nih.gov/pmc/articles/PMC7132018/

54. Møller S, Bendtsen F. The pathophysiology of arterial vasodilatation and hyperdynamic circulation in cirrhosis. Liver International [Internet]. 2018 [cited July 3, 2023];38(4):570-80. Available from: https://onlinelibrary.wiley.com/doi/abs/10.1111/liv.13589

55. Sahay M, Sahay R. Hyponatremia: A practical approach. Indian J

Endocrinol Metab [Internet]. 2014 [cited 3 July 2023];18(6):760-71. Available from: https://www.ncbi.nlm.nih.gov/pmc/articles/PMC4192979/

56. Ospina LLG, Laverde JLG, Tapia JAA, Cahuasquí JPO. Hyponatremia and hepatorenal syndrome. RECIMUNDO [Internet]. July 11, 2020 [cited July 3, 2023];4(3):102-17. Available from: https://recimundo.com/index.php/es/article/view/854

57. de Mattos ÂZ, Simonetto DA, Terra C, Farias AQ, Bittencourt PL, Pase THS, et al. Albumin administration in patients with cirrhosis: Current role and novel perspectives. World J Gastroenterol [Internet]. September 7, 2022 [cited July 3, 2023];28(33):4773-86. Available from: https://www.ncbi.nlm.nih.gov/pmc/articles/PMC9476855/

58. Baek SH, Jo YH, Ahn S, Medina-Liabres K, Oh YK, Lee JB, et al. Risk of Overcorrection in Rapid Intermittent Bolus vs Slow Continuous Infusion Therapies of Hypertonic Saline for Patients With Symptomatic Hyponatremia. JAMA Intern Med [Internet]. January 2021 [cited 2023 July 3];181(1):1-12. Available from: https://www.ncbi.nlm.nih.gov/pmc/articles/PMC7589081/

59. Berl T, Quittnat-Pelletier F, Verbalis JG, Schrier RW, Bichet DG, Ouyang J, et al. Oral Tolvaptan Is Safe and Effective in Chronic Hyponatremia. J Am Soc Nephrol [Internet]. April 2010 [cited 3 July 2023];21(4):705-12. Available from: https://www.ncbi.nlm.nih.gov/pmc/articles/PMC2844305/

60. Sequera PO de, Álcazar Arroyo R, Albalate Ramón M. Nefrología al Día. 2021 [cited 1 August 2023]. Potassium disorders. Hypokalaemia. Hyperkalaemia | Nephrology Today. Available at: http://www.nefrologiaaldia.org/es-articulo-potassium-disorders-potassium-hypokalaemia-hyperkalaemia-383

61. Younes R, Caviglia GP, Govaere O, Rosso C, Armandi A, Sanavia T, et al. Long-term outcomes and predictive ability of non-invasive scoring systems in patients with non-alcoholic fatty liver disease. J Hepatol. Oct 2021;75(4):786-94.

62. Defás Zambrano GE, Mogro Espinoza MA. Hyponatremia as a factor related to mortality in patients with liver cirrhosis hospitalized at Hospital Teodoro Maldonado Carbo during 2018-2019. May 1, 2021 [cited August 1, 2023]; Available from: http://repositorio.ucsg.edu.ec/handle/3317/16695

63. G S, C P, C A, Ms S, S M. Prevalence of hyponatremia in chronic liver disease patients and it's correlation with the severity of the disease. J Assoc Physicians India. April 2022;70(4):11-2.

64. Bhandari A, Chaudhary A. Hyponatremia in Chronic Liver Disease among Patients Presenting to a Tertiary Care Hospital: A Descriptive Cross-sectional

Study. JNMA J Nepal Med Assoc [Internet]. December 2021 [cited 1 August 2023];59(244):1225-8. Available from:
https://www.ncbi.nlm.nih.gov/pmc/articles/PMC9200023/
65. Yperti MJ, Ordoñez M. Prevalence and factors associated with hyponatremia in older adults from 2016 to 2018, at Hospital Alcívar. Revista Actas Médicas [Internet]. 2023;31(1):9. Available at:
https://issuu.com/hospitalalcivar2/docs/revista_actas_medicas_31_vol_1/s/13585949
66. Bashir S, Pervaiz A, Khan HA, Tahir HM, Hasham A, Hafeez MS, et al. Frequency of Hyponatremia in Patients with Hepatic Encephalopathy at a tertiary care hospital. 2019;13(2):306-8. Available at:
https://pjmhsonline.com/2019/april_june/pdf/306.pdf

ANNEX 1. RESULTS OF TABLES

Table 4. Patient characteristics according to sex, age, drugs and length of hospital stay

Sex	Frequency	%
Male	55	49,5%
Female	56	50,5%
Total	111	100,0%
Age	Frequency	%
30 - 50	5	4,5%
51 - 70	72	64,9%
71 - 91	34	30,6%
Total	111	100,0%
Use of drugs (diuretics)	Frequency	%
Yes	70	63,1%
No	41	36,9%
Total	111	100,0%
Hospital stay	Frequency	%
1 - 15 days	80	72,1%
16 - 30 days	25	22,5%
31 - 46 days	6	5,4%
Total	111	100,0%

Source: Internal data from Hospital General del Norte de Guayaquil IESS Los Ceibos Prepared by: Authors.

Prevalence of degrees of hyponatraemia in patients with liver cirrhosis.

Degrees of hyponatremia	Number of cases	Patients with liver cirrhosis (same period)	Prevalence	
Slight	75		0,2373	23,7%
Moderate	32	316	0,1013	10,1%
Severe	4		0,0127	1,3%
Total	111		0,3513	35,1%

Source: Internal data from the Hospital General del Norte de Guayaquil IESS Los Ceibos. Prepared by: Authors.

Relationship between the degree of hyponatraemia and comorbidities associated with liver cirrhosis.

Associated comorbidities		Degrees of hyponatremia			Total	P-value
		Slight	Moderate	Severe		
Arterial hypertension						0,063
No	Count	37	8	2	47	
	% of total	33,3%	7,2%	1,8%	42,3%	
Yes	Count	38	24	2	64	
	% of total	34,2%	21,6%	1,8%	57,7%	
Total	Count	75	32	4	111	
	% of total	67,6%	28,8%	3,6%	100,0%	
Diabetes Mellitus						0,432
No	Count	43	14	2	59	
	% of total	38,7%	12,6%	1,8%	53,2%	
Yes	Count	32	18	2	52	
	% of total	28,8%	16,2%	1,8%	46,8%	
Total	Count	75	32	4	111	
	% of total	67,6%	28,8%	3,6%	100,0%	
Chronic kidney disease						0,263
No	Count	62	23	4	89	
	% of total	55,9%	20,7%	3,6%	80,2%	
Yes	Count	13	9	0	22	
	% of total	11,7%	8,1%	0,0%	19,8%	
Total	Count	75	32	4	111	
	% of total	67,6%	28,8%	3,6%	100,0%	
Cancer						0,049
No	Count	67	23	4	94	
	% of total	60,4%	20,7%	3,6%	84,7%	
Yes	Count	8	9	0	17	
	% of total	7,2%	8,1%	0,0%	15,3%	
Total	Count	75	32	4	111	
	% of total	67,6%	28,8%	3,6%	100,0%	
Infectious (TB)						0,337
No	Count	74	30	4	108	
	% of total	66,7%	27,0%	3,6%	97,3%	
Yes	Count	1	2	0	3	
	% of total	0,9%	1,8%	0,0%	2,7%	
Total	Count	75	32	4	111	
	% of total	67,6%	28,8%	3,6%	100,0%	

Source: Internal data from Hospital General del Norte de Guayaquil IESS Los Ceibos. Prepared by: Authors.

Table 7. Severity of cirrhosis and the degree of hyponatremia

Child-Pugh scale		Degrees of hyponatremia			Total	P-value
		Slight	Moderate	Severe		
Severity of cirrhosis						0,256
A	Count	15	4	1	20	
	% of total	13,5%	3,6%	0,9%	18,0%	
B	Count	35	10	2	47	
	% of total	31,5%	9,0%	1,8%	42,3%	
C	Count	25	18	1	44	
	% of total	22,5%	16,2%	0,9%	39,6%	
Total	Count	75	32	4	111	
	% of total	67,6%	28,8%	3,6%	100,0%	

Source: Internal data from Hospital General del Norte de Guayaquil IESS Los Ceibos Prepared by: Authors.

Table 8. Distribution of the degree of hyponatraemia according to the stage of cirrhosis

Clinical stage of cirrhosis		Degrees of hyponatremia			Total	P-value
		Slight	Moderate	Severe		
Stage of cirrhosis						0,213
Unbalanced	Count	57	29	3	89	
	% of total	51,4%	26,1%	2,7%	80,2%	
Compensated	Count	18	3	1	22	
	% of total	16,2%	2,7%	0,9%	19,8%	
Total	Count	75	32	4	111	
	% of total	67,6%	28,8%	3,6%	100,0%	

Source: Internal data from Hospital General del Norte de Guayaquil IESS Los Ceibos Prepared by: Authors

Table 9. Relationship between the degree of hyponatraemia and the most common complications in patients with liver cirrhosis

Associated comorbidities		Degrees of hyponatremia			Total	P-value
		Slight	Moderate	Severe		
Hepatic encephalopathy						0,071
0	Count	30	7	0	37	
	% of total	27,0%	6,3%	0,0%	33,3%	
1	Count	16	6	3	25	
	% of total	14,4%	5,4%	2,7%	22,5%	
2	Count	18	12	1	31	
	% of total	16,2%	10,8%	0,9%	27,9%	
3	Count	11	7	0	18	
	% of total	9,9%	6,3%	0,0%	16,2%	
4	Count	0	0	0	0	
	% of total	0,0%	0,0%	0,0%	0,0%	
Total	Count	75	32	4	111	
	% of total	67,6%	28,8%	3,6%	100,0%	
Oesophageal varices						0,344
No	Count	30	17	1	48	
	% of total	27,0%	15,3%	0,9%	43,2%	
Yes	Count	45	15	3	63	
	% of total	40,5%	13,5%	2,7%	56,8%	
Total	Count	75	32	4	111	
	% of total	67,6%	28,8%	3,6%	100,0%	
Non-variceal upper gastrointestinal haemorrhage (NAUH)						0,032
No	Count	49	20	0	69	
	% of total	44,1%	18,0%	0,0%	62,2%	
Yes	Count	26	12	4	42	
	% of total	23,4%	10,8%	3,6%	37,8%	
Total	Count	75	32	4	111	
	% of total	67,6%	28,8%	3,6%	100,0%	
Jaundice						0,124
No	Count	64	24	2	90	
	% of total	57,7%	21,6%	1,8%	81,1%	
Yes	Count	11	8	2	21	
	% of total	9,9%	7,2%	1,8%	18,9%	
Total	Count	75	32	4	111	
	% of total	67,6%	28,8%	3,6%	100,0%	
Ascites						0,957
No	Count	32	14	2	48	
	% of total	28,8%	12,6%	1,8%	43,2%	

Yes	Count	43	18	2	63	
	% of total	38,7%	16,2%	1,8%	56,8%	
Total	Count	75	32	4	111	
	% of total	67,6%	28,8%	3,6%	100,0%	

Source: Internal data from Hospital General del Norte de Guayaquil IESS Ceibos Prepared by: Authors

Table 10. Crosstabulation of variables: Age and sex

Variable		Sex		Total	P-value
		Female	Male		
Age					0,909
30 - 50	Count	3	2	5	
	% of total	2,7%	1,8%	4,5%	
51 - 70	Count	36	36	72	
	% of total	32,4%	32,4%	64,9%	
71 - 91	Count	17	17	34	
	% of total	15,3%	15,3%	30,6%	
Total	Count	56	55	111	
	% of total	50,5%	49,5%	100,0%	

Source: Internal data from Hospital General del Norte de Guayaquil IESS Los Ceibos Prepared by: Authors

Table 11. Crosstabulation of variables, age, sex and degrees of hyponatremia

Variables		Degrees of hyponatremia			Total	P-value
		Slight	Moderate	Severe		
Sex						0,889
Female	Count	39	15	2	56	
	% of total	35,1%	13,5%	1,8%	50,5%	
Male	Count	36	17	2	55	
	% of total	32,4%	15,3%	1,8%	49,5%	
Total	Count	75	32	4	111	
	% of total	67,6%	28,8%	3,6%	100,0%	
Age						0,209
30 - 50	Count	4	0	1	5	
	% of total	3,6%	0,0%	0,9%	4,5%	
51 - 70	Count	47	23	2	72	
	% of total	42,3%	20,7%	1,8%	64,9%	
71 - 91	Count	24	9	1	34	
	% of total	21,6%	8,1%	0,9%	30,6%	
Total	Count	75	32	4	111	
	% of total	67,6%	28,8%	3,6%	100,0%	

Source: Internal data from Hospital General del Norte de Guayaquil IESS Los Ceibos Prepared by: Authors

Crosstabulation of variables, age, sex and clinical stage of cirrhosis.

Variables		Clinical stage of cirrhosis		Total	P-value
		Unbalanced	Compensated		
Sex					0,365
Female	Count	43	13	56	
	% of total	38,7%	11,7%	50,5%	
Male	Count	46	9	55	
	% of total	41,4%	8,1%	49,5%	
Total	Count	89	22	111	
	% of total	80,2%	19,8%	100,0%	
Age					0,002
30 - 50	Count	1	4	5	
	% of total	0,9%	3,6%	4,5%	
51 - 70	Count	61	11	72	
	% of total	55,0%	9,9%	64,9%	
71 - 91	Count	27	7	34	
	% of total	24,3%	6,3%	30,6%	
Total	Count	89	22	111	
	% of total	80,2%	19,8%	100,0%	

Source: Internal data from Hospital General del Norte de Guayaquil IESS Los Ceibos Prepared by: Authors

Table 13. Cross-tabulation of variables, sex and complications of liver cirrhosis

Variable		Sex		Total	P-value
		Female	Male		
Hepatic encephalopathy					0,440
0	Count	22	15	37	
	% of total	19,8%	13,5%	33,3%	
1	Count	11	14	25	
	% of total	9,9%	12,6%	22,5%	
2	Count	13	18	31	
	% of total	11,7%	16,2%	27,9%	
3	Count	10	8	18	
	% of total	9,0%	7,2%	16,2%	
4	Count	0	0	0	
	% of total	0,0%	0,0%	0,0%	
Total	Count	56	55	111	
	% of total	50,5%	49,5%	100,0%	
Oesophageal varices					0,046
No	Count	19	29	48	
	% of total	17,1%	26,1%	43,2%	

Yes	Count	37	26	63	
	% of total	33,3%	23,4%	56,8%	
Total	Count	56	55	111	
	% of total	50,5%	49,5%	100,0%	
Non-variceal upper gastrointestinal haemorrhage (NAUH)					0,478
No	Count	33	36	69	
	% of total	29,7%	32,4%	62,2%	
Yes	Count	23	19	42	
	% of total	20,7%	17,1%	37,8%	
Total	Count	56	55	111	
	% of total	50,5%	49,5%	100,0%	
Jaundice					0,440
No	Count	47	43	90	
	% of total	42,3%	38,7%	81,1%	
Yes	Count	9	12	21	
	% of total	8,1%	10,8%	18,9%	
Total	Count	56	55	111	
	% of total	50,5%	49,5%	100,0%	
Ascites					0,494
No	Count	26	22	48	
	% of total	23,4%	19,8%	43,2%	
Yes	Count	30	33	63	
	% of total	27,0%	29,7%	56,8%	
Total	Count	56	55	111	
	% of total	50,5%	49,5%	100,0%	

Source: Internal data from the Hospital General del Norte de Guayaquil IESS Los Ceibos. Prepared by: Authors

Table 14. Cross-tabulation of variables, age and complications of liver cirrhosis

Variable		Age			Total	P-value
		30 - 50	51 - 70	71 - 91		
Hepatic encephalopathy						0,333
0	Count	3	23	11	37	
	% of total	2,7%	20,7%	9,9%	33,3%	
1	Count	2	14	9	25	
	% of total	1,8%	12,6%	8,1%	22,5%	
2	Count	0	20	11	31	
	% of total	0,0%	18,0%	9,9%	27,9%	
3	Count	0	15	3	18	
	% of total	0,0%	13,5%	2,7%	16,2%	

4	Count	0	0	0	0	
	% of total	0,0%	0,0%	0,0%	0,0%	
Total	Count	5	72	34	111	
	% of total	4,5%	64,9%	30,6%	100,0%	
Oesophageal varices						0,940
No	Count	2	32	14	48	
	% of total	1,8%	28,8%	12,6%	43,2%	
Yes	Count	3	40	20	63	
	% of total	2,7%	36,0%	18,0%	56,8%	
Total	Count	5	72	34	111	
	% of total	4,5%	64,9%	30,6%	100,0%	
Non-variceal upper gastrointestinal haemorrhage (NAUH)						0,566
No	Count	2	46	21	69	
	% of total	1,8%	41,4%	18,9%	62,2%	
Yes	Count	3	26	13	42	
	% of total	2,7%	23,4%	11,7%	37,8%	
Total	Count	5	72	34	111	
	% of total	4,5%	64,9%	30,6%	100,0%	
Jaundice						0,752
No	Count	4	57	29	90	
	% of total	3,6%	51,4%	26,1%	81,1%	
Yes	Count	1	15	5	21	
	% of total	0,9%	13,5%	4,5%	18,9%	
Total	Count	5	72	34	111	
	% of total	4,5%	64,9%	30,6%	100,0%	
Ascites						0,597
No	Count	3	29	16	48	
	% of total	2,7%	26,1%	14,4%	43,2%	
Yes	Count	2	43	18	63	
	% of total	1,8%	38,7%	16,2%	56,8%	
Total	Count	5	72	34	111	
	% of total	4,5%	64,9%	30,6%	100,0%	

Source: Internal data from Hospital General del Norte de Guayaquil IESS Los Ceibos Prepared by: Authors

ANNEX 2. RESULTS OF GRAPHS

Figure 4. Recognition of the sample

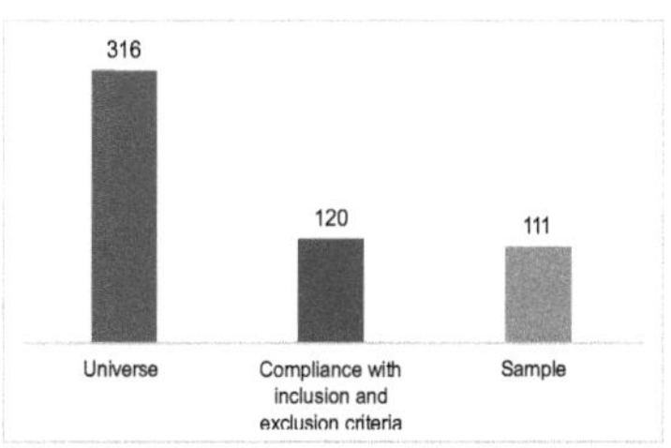

Figure 5. Sex of patients in the study

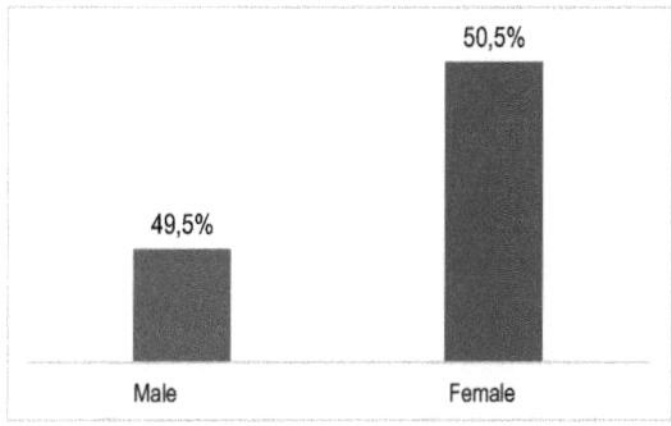

Figure 6. Use of drugs (diuretics) in the study population

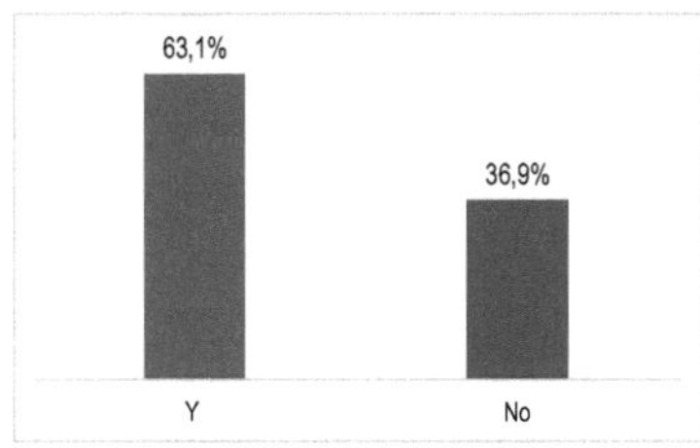

Graph 7. Hospital stay within the study

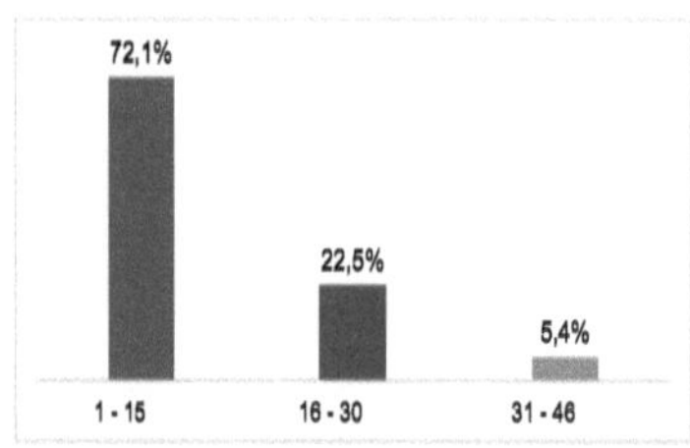

Graph 8. Degrees of hyponatremia in the study population

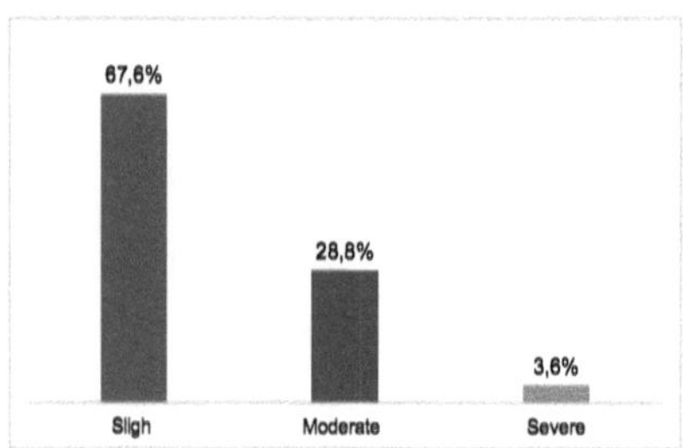

Figure 9. Comorbidities present and degrees of hyponatremia

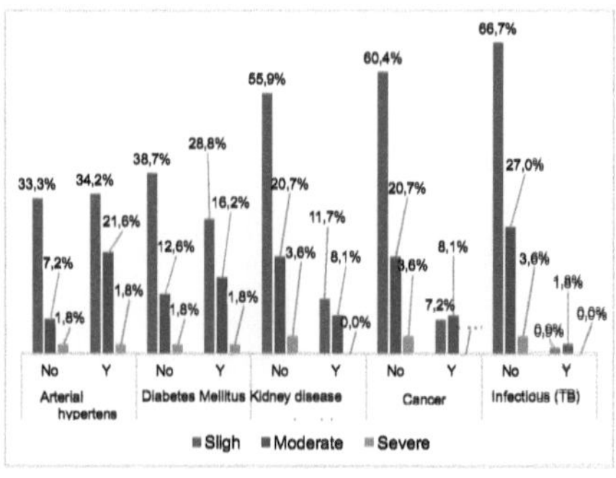

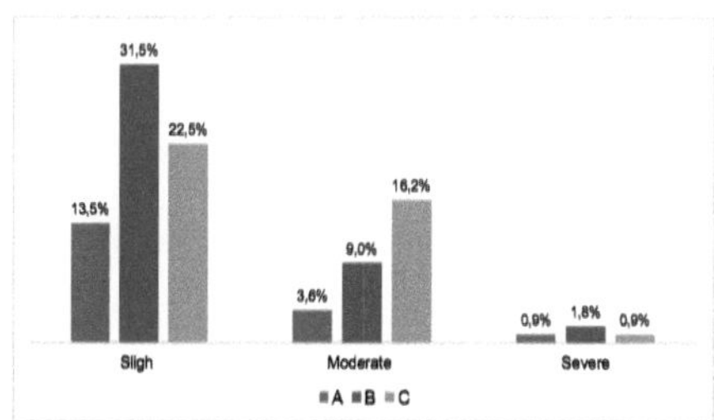

Figure 11. Clinical stage of cirrhosis and degrees of hyponatremia

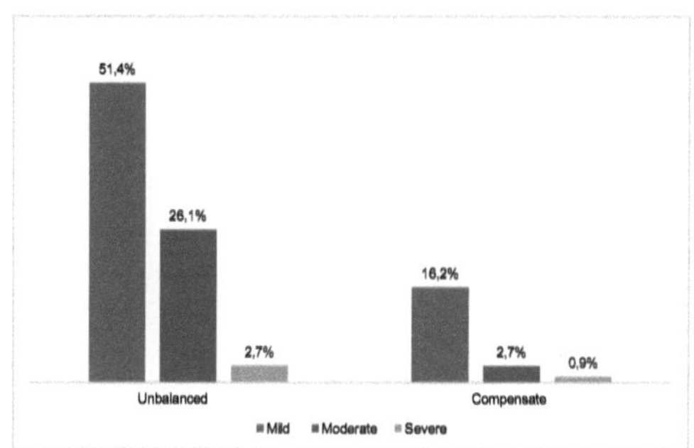

Figure 12. Complications and degrees of hyponatraemia

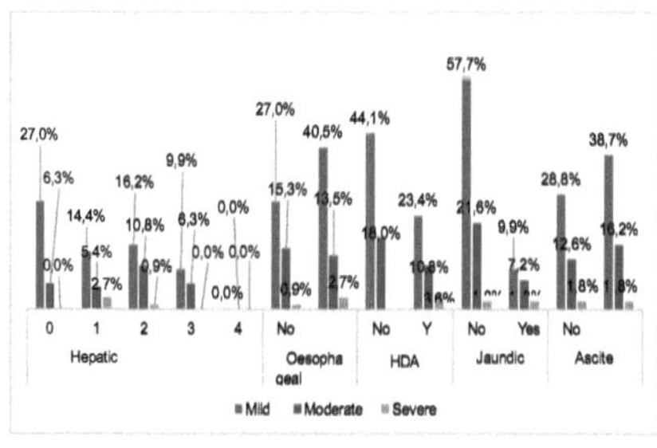

Graph 13. Relationship between age and sex of the population studied.

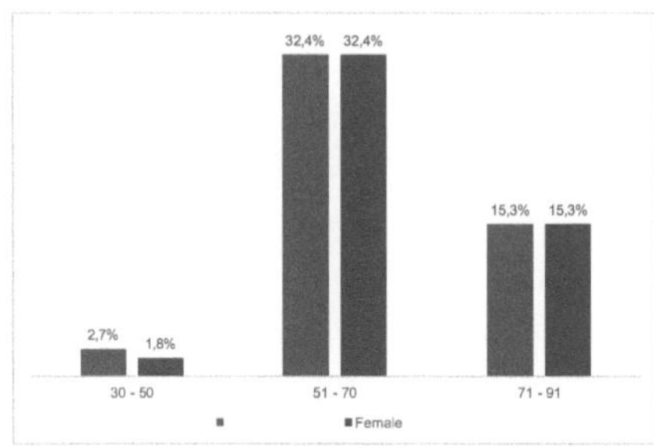

Figure 14. Relationship between age, sex and degrees of hyponatremia

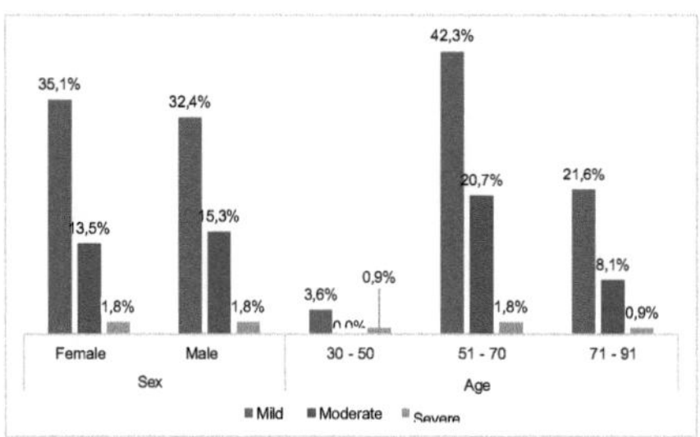

Figure 15. Relationship between age, sex and clinical stage of cirrhosis

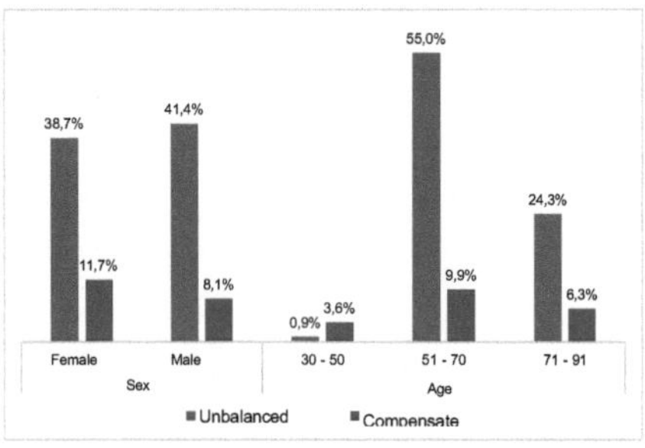

Graph 16. Relationship between sex and most frequent complications in the patients under study.

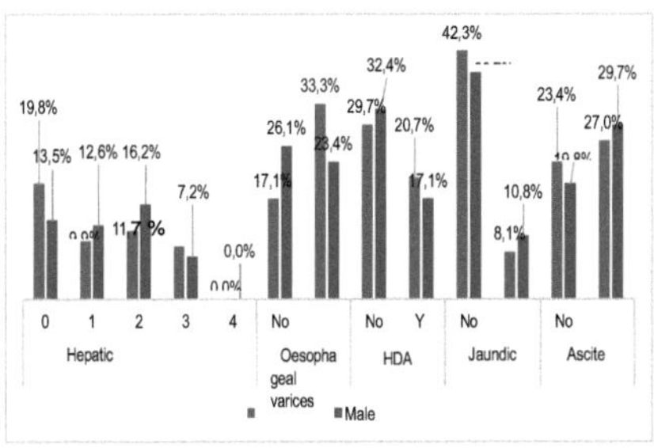

Figure 17. Relationship between age and complications of liver cirrhosis

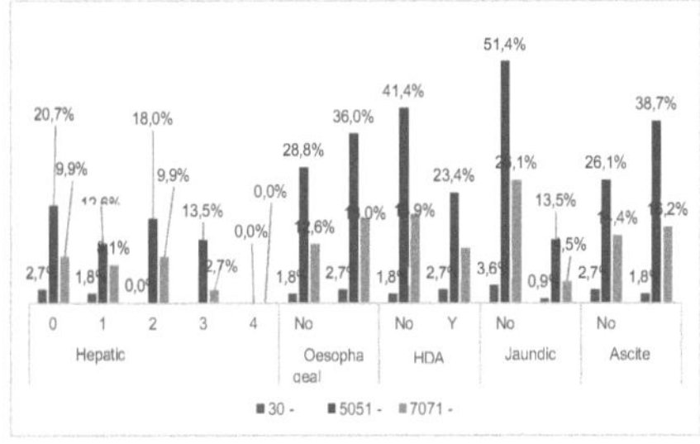

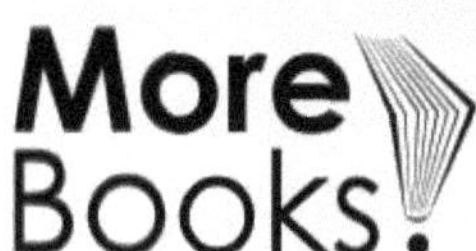

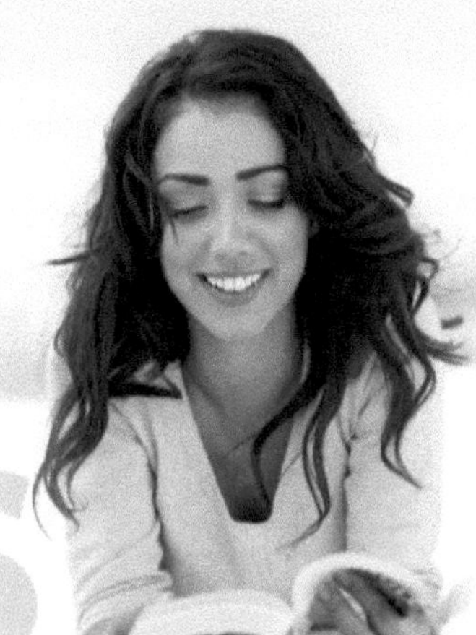

yes
I want morebooks!

Buy your books fast and straightforward online - at one of world's fastest growing online book stores! Environmentally sound due to Print-on-Demand technologies.

Buy your books online at
www.morebooks.shop

Kaufen Sie Ihre Bücher schnell und unkompliziert online – auf einer der am schnellsten wachsenden Buchhandelsplattformen weltweit! Dank Print-On-Demand umwelt- und ressourcenschonend produziert.

Bücher schneller online kaufen
www.morebooks.shop

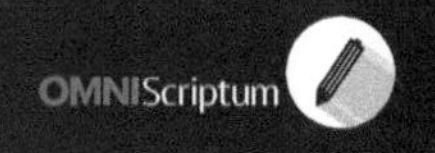

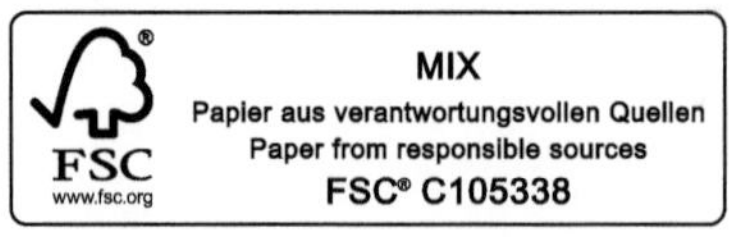

Printed by Books on Demand GmbH, Norderstedt / Germany